AFRICAN DANCE
WITH PASSION

First Edition

By Kukuwa Kyereboah-Nuamah
George Mason University

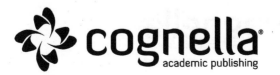

Bassim Hamadeh, CEO and Publisher
Michael Simpson, Vice President of Acquisitions
Jamie Giganti, Managing Editor
Jess Busch, Graphic Design Supervisor
Amy Stone, Acquisitions Editor
Mirasol Enriquez, Project Editor
Luiz Ferreira, Senior Licensing Specialist

ISBN: 978-1-63487-035-1 (pbk)/ 978-1-63487-036-8 (br)

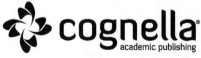

academic publishing

www.cognella.com   800-200-3908

CONTENTS

Chapter 1: Introduction to African Dance   1

Chapter 2: Mind-Body Preparation for Dance Class   29

Chapter 3: Health and Safety Attributes of Dance   39

Chapter 4: Learning and Performing the Basics of
          African Dance   61

Chapter 5: Foundations of African Dance Techniques   93

Chapter 6: Template for African Dances Taught in Class 135

Chapter 7: History of African Dance Styles   163

ACKNOWLEDGMENTS

First of all, I would like to thank Almighty God, my mentor, who put the right people in my path to make this book happen. I also wish to express my sincere gratitude and appreciation to my lovely sister, Bernice Taylor, who took time off to research and help me expand my chapters, and for her valuable input of beautiful writing. A zillion thanks also goes out to Tom Johnson, who assisted me in the editing, proofreading, and further research, along with his love of writing, to complete this book. Thanks to all those who provided support and encouragement throughout my writing.

Above all to, my late mother and my living father for such a disciplined upbringing I am grateful for and which I will always cherish.

Thanks to my Cognella Publishers Sarah Wheeler, Chelsey Rogers, Jennifer Levin, Amy Stone, and Ivey Preston, who worked alongside me to finish this book. Thanks to Jess Busch for patiently working with me to get the beautiful and rightful cover for my book.

Being a "night owl," I credit my late-night hours to the finish of this book, as those were the quietest times of my day that allowed me to do my writing. I believe that my passion for dance, particularly African dance, has enabled me to write and share this book. Sharing such passion with you through this book has been a blessing for me, because my burning desire for teaching people to stay healthy and fit through my dancing can now be found through my books.

I dedicate this book solely to my two daughters, Cassandra Mame Ekua Nuamah and Samantha Nana Esi Nuamah, whom I believe were born to dance like I was when I was born. Dancing runs deep within my family. I grew up knowing my great grandmother, my grandmother, and my mother as fabulous dancers who would never stop dancing until the music stopped. I have grown up with the same passion in my heart and can't seem to stop "moving my boombsey" forever. All my six siblings and all my 13 nieces and nephews love to dance at any given occasion, as this runs deep in our entire family.

I pray that my book will open a brand-new desire of dancing in your life and allow you to see what the benefits of African dancing can do for you.

As my dance slogan always goes … start reading, so you can "move your boombsey" with me!

Thank you for buying my book and for taking the time to read it.

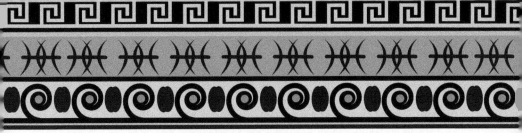

Chapter 1

INTRODUCTION TO AFRICAN DANCE

African dancing is an experience of the soul that puts a smile on everyone's face and a challenge in their step. It changes the lives of many who have never taken it before, from young to old, adults to minors, novice to expert. African dance is exciting, exhilarating, intriguing, puts one in high spirits, and piques one's interest all the way through the dance. It is challenging, yet inviting. It will have you moving in every direction and moving muscles you didn't even know you had. It will allow you to express yourself and come out of your comfort zone in an amazing way.

As Welsh put it, "Dance in Africa is a holistic part of society. It is not just truncated or separated as an entity in and of itself. Dance is used to facilitate all phenomena in most African societies. [It] developed as an essential, functional part of life."

There are a wide array of dances in Africa, including ceremonial dances, war dances, royal dances, and rites of passage. Dancing is not just reserved for happy times, but also for sad occasions. It is customary, for instance, to celebrate a person's life with dancing after they are buried. Some African cultures believe there is a time for everything, and that joy and celebration should follow the weeping and lamentation. Although this may seem strange to some Western cultures, this is acceptable and required.

When learning African dance, you will realize it entails many elements, including orientation toward the Earth, **polyrhythms**, musicality, and body isolations that combine to comprise a dance in its entirety. You will learn to move your head and neck, your legs and feet, your arms, and your torso and pelvis in rhythm with drums in isolation, and then combined, to complete a dance movement.

To quote Nettleford, "Africa and Africans have not been short on the complexity of the creative process and the sustainability of what the human being anywhere can produce from the individual and collective creative imagination and intellect."

DEFINING AFRICAN DANCE

Africa is a continent that is about three times the size of the United States, made up of about 56 countries and their capitals and numerous languages and dialects. It is ethnically and culturally the most diverse continent on the planet. The term **tribe** will be used throughout this book. Tribe is a word that has been utilized throughout history and across cultures, from the Twelve Tribes of Israel, to Native American tribes, to the hippie tribes of the 1960s.

Today, tribes play an integral part in the lives of the African people. Each region in a particular country is made up of several tribes. In Ghana alone, which is populated by about 20 million people, there are about 58 tribes, and each tribe speaks its own language or dialect. So one can only imagine the magnitude of tribes and languages of the people of Africa. African dance is the foundation of the continent on a large scale. The music of Africa from all over the different regions of the continent, made up of numerous tribes, is the true language of Africa. No matter which region or tribe one comes from, when Africans get together and the music and dance are in motion, it becomes one big celebration. This sort of party lasts hours on end and can continue from one day to the next for about three days in a row at times. African dance allows its people to express themselves profoundly in ways that supersede an actual language. African dance is certainly unlike other genres of dance. Its connectivity to music greatly portrays its outstanding difference from any other genre of dance.

African dance tells a story in many cases. You will learn that a dance can relate a life event, define a ceremony, or convey a belief. In your African dance class, you will learn, among others, a dance of warriors and a dance of freedom from oppression, as well as a coming-of-age dance. Your body will move in ways that are foreign to it, yet you will appreciate the essence of what is being conveyed when you have learned the dance and its accompanying story. Soon, the call of *woso woso* will mean "shake it" to you, as opposed to just some foreign **Akan** words.

The technique of African dance is formulated by the emotions, sentiments, and beliefs of the dancer. The body speaks the language of dance as the dancers express their emotions through the dances and move to the rhythm of the drums with all of their body, mind, and spirit, as if they have no bones in their bodies. Addressing a person by saying they dance as if they had no bones in their body is one of the highest African dance compliments. Students who hear the instructor give this compliment can be assured they are executing the dances as an African.

African Dance Today

African dance has sustained the genuineness of the origination of dances that were passed down from generation to generation. In the past, the dances were taught by sight and not by word, as reading and writing were not taught then. Today, it is still taught a majority of the time by sight, as this method has proven to work for ages. The student has to keep their eye on the teacher and watch her movements, synchronized to the drums being played by the drummers. Counting is not the norm, as in teaching dance today. The student is taught to pay attention and listen attentively to the drums played in order to feel the beat and to start dancing as the teacher does on the downbeat of the drum. Some of the dance forms that are being taught in our schools today are derived directly from African dances. Jazz, modern jazz, hip-hop, krumping, popping, stepping, and break dancing are among the most common.

As stated in *Zimbabwe Dance*, "The colonial and post-colonial eras robbed African people worldwide of much essential information on traditional African cultures. Now that void is gradually being filled.

Studies of traditional African dances have opened a uniquely pan-
oramic window into those traditional societies where the dance itself
stands as an aesthetic ledger that chronicles as well as facilitates the
social life of the community."

Gender and African Dance

Even in some dances where females and males dance together, there
are some guidelines about how the two genders should relate. In some
courtship dances like Neely of the Karimojong people of northeastern
Uganda, body contact among dancing partners is prohibited until later
in the dance. However, in most parts of Africa and Western culture,
African dance is open to males and females. In Ghana, both genders
dance and drum, so both are encouraged to take the class for the
experience. This book will open the minds of males as well as females
that African dance is for everyone. Since some African ceremonies are
specific to certain genders, such as rites of passage, some dances are
traditionally only performed by males or females. However, at George
Mason University, all dances are taught to all students, despite gender.
This gives the student the experience of learning all the dances.

Benefits of African Dance for Students

First of all, rhythm for a dancer is felt in the body before heard; this
is what enables the dancer to move, synchronized with the beat.
Africans term that a Mind, Body, Spirit experience. Benefits of African
dance are the flexibility one gets in their body and muscles, while
toning, firming and losing body fat. African dances work every part
of the body because the movements are so intense. From the head
to the toes, there is no part of the body that is not involved in the
dances. The movements use both the large and small muscle groups
in the body, which is a great benefit to the dancer. The student will
experience the benefits of the body right away in this class such as
weight loss due to the intensity of the dance movements. The dances
will have the students' minds take them on a journey to a particular
African country in every class, due to the story of the dance that
paints the vivid picture. The dances are mostly typically cultural and

set in a village atmosphere, which gives the student the actual feel of being there via the dances.

There are many places in Africa where people live to be over 80, 90, and 100 years of age in the villages, where lifestyles come from the resources of nature derived from Mother Earth. Much of research shows that we all came out of Africa. The civilization in Africa, then, is perhaps the oldest in the world. The tribal cultures have developed many ways of coping with illness and disease and extending the life spans of its people. In our present world, people are not living healthy lifestyles to make it to age 100; people are hardly enjoying a good quality of life in their 70s and 80s. As a society, we need to change our habits and turn things around for our own benefit. Learning how to eat, drink, exercise, and relax properly will enable us to live both longer and healthier lives.

Studying African Dance as an Academic Subject

Why Study African Dance?

One should study African dance to gain the appreciation of the dance, its format, meaning, ethnicity, culture, and benefits. The emotional aspect of African dance allows the student to feel the depth of the dance, especially when they are told the story behind the dance. The physical aspect of the dance enables the student to experience the true meaning of the culture of the people. The intellectual aspect of the dance moves the student from one level to another, which is even higher, allowing them to attain the knowledge behind the dance.

African dances are learned to accomplish the following:

- To acquaint oneself with the African ritualistic dance traditions revolving around everyday life, as well as ongoing life processes in the African communities
- To gain insight into the "interconnectedness, difference, and diversity of a global society" through learning the societal norms of African cultures and how they fit into or stand out from Western culture, as well as a direct contrast of the African cultures themselves
- To devise analytical, practical, or creative responses to global problems or issues, becoming familiar with the histories (apart-

heid, etc.) that influenced African dances as a way of communicating these stories

The First Class

The first time a student walks into an African dance class, they are a bit nervous, not necessarily knowing what to expect by the description of the class. A method of easing students into this type of class is to start by having them all in a classroom circle, welcoming them, and telling them a bit about the instructor's background. Once the students' attention is obtained, the instructor goes around the circle asking every student to tell the whole class their name and their parental background. This method allows everyone to open up and ease up a bit, plus it gives the instructor an idea of the various backgrounds in the class. First things first: the instructor gives students an overview of African culture and dance (which can be found in Chapters 2 and 7).

A typical class will include a mixture of students, some of whom are dance majors, others who have never taken dance before, and others who have taken different genres of dance, but not yet African. Even those who have taken African dance before find it a challenge. This challenge is a positive one that grooms each student. When you take this fun class, it will make you feel confident and disciplined, and it will build your stamina regardless of your level. You might commence the class not knowing coordination, rhythm, or beat, but by the end of the semester, the challenge will prove to be a truly rewarding experience for you.

Student Concerns

Many students think they know what difficulties to expect. Every excuse in the book is given. "Professor, I am not a dancer." "Professor, I really cannot dance; I have two left feet." "Professor, I'm Irish, and I am not that flexible." "Professor, I have never danced in my life before, so I'm not sure what I can do." This is to be expected, as the syllabus lets students know what the course study will be, even before class starts. Students all feel the fun of the class because the instructor conveys the thought that effort is the key to success. The expectation for students is that if you put in the effort despite your excuses, you will overcome it all and end up doing your very best. The instructor will encourage each student and compliment their efforts in front of the other students, allowing them to feel more confident in taking the class.

Taking an African dance class for the first time can be exciting, exhilarating, and challenging, all at the same time. Whatever concerns students have, as soon as the drums are played and the rhythm sounds throughout the class, they can't wait to move their **boombseys**. The class lasts about an hour and a half, and students are expected to dance for at most 60 minutes out of the 90. However, one of the things students enjoy most is that time becomes of no essence to them.

African dance can be a whole new world to anyone who does not really know Africa. This book will cover all grounds to educate the beginner, intermediate or advance person on African dance. No particular skills are needed.

AFRICAN DANCE CLASS STRUCTURE

Story-Time Circle

Before a new dance is taught, the instructor will get the class back into the story-time circle, created at the beginning of the semester. The beginning of every class starts out with the circle, attendance, and story time, which gives each student a relaxed feeling. Students then get into the African line (mentioned in Chapter 2), and the instructor begins to teach them the breakdown of the dance moves for that particular dance. This method breaks the ice for students.

The Warm-Up

There certainly has to be a warm-up phase for African dance. Students need to warm up their muscles from the head, to the torso, to the hips, to the boombseys, to the arms and legs. African dance is a total body workout, so all small and large muscles are used in every dance. The class warms up in a lineup of two rows that goes around the room to the beat of the drums at a slow pace until all limbs are warmed up, ready for dance. This takes about 15 minutes.

The Buildup Section

Students stay in the lineup row after the warm-up and begin to escalate their movements to the drums, which pick up in tempo for a buildup toward the peak. This is necessary to help build stamina for the students who usually come to class out of shape. The buildup section of the dance class lasts for about another 15 minutes. The best part is each student feels they are in shape by the end of the semester.

Learning the Dance

Students love learning the dances in a long line as the drummer plays for them to move down the lines. The instructor will repeat all break-downs for eight counts and then four, so they have plenty of practice on each movement. The instructor will perform this sequence for every dance students need to learn, and this gives them the necessary preparedness. Instructors will use the 10–12 weeks out of the 14 weeks to teach all 10 dances. Students will be paired up with a buddy with whom they can practice the dances, and this helps them immensely. Weeks 12–13 will be used to go over all the ten dances and prepare the students for finals.

The Peak Section

The peak section is the ultimate stamina upsurge for the students because the drums play faster and louder, encouraging and urging the students on to move even more vibrantly. This section is both the fun and the hard parts for students because you see them tired, but laughing or smiling because they are still having fun. This is the "move your boombsey" section that all the students love to hate, because it lasts even longer, for about 20 to 25 minutes. It is guaranteed to have everyone sweating.

The Cooldown

Then comes the cooldown, which students really love after all the sweating and hard work they have done. The drums once again begin to slow down in pace and tempo to enable the students to lessen their movements and stretch their muscles out to avoid any aftermath muscle pain. Students go through a cooldown phase at every class, as this is a necessity in dance. This section is about ten minutes long, and it ends with the students on their knees tapping the floor along with the beat of the drummer, indicating their gratitude.

SPECIFICS OF ACADEMIC AFRICAN DANCE

Music and the Musicians for Dance

A live drummer plays music for an African dance class. To give the class the authenticity of African dance, a live drummer makes the class come to life with the drumbeats and rhythms. While not all African dances use only drums, in class, the drummer takes his lead from the teacher, and the two work hand in hand to set the mood of the class. All dances are first played at a slow pace, allowing students to grasp the moves at their own pace; then the drummer speeds up the tempo a few beats more, engaging students into more movements until they are ready to move full speed.

Welsh articulated the relationship between dancing and drumming like this: "Contextually, dancing and drumming are the same. Although perceived differently they both emanate from the same foundation, namely rhythm." Locke put it this way: "Dancers provide a crucial source of inspiration for the improvising musician. In Gahu, musical form is a product of choreography."

The Dance Studio

The dance studio must be spacious and well lighted. Ventilation is very important, as the students will be sweating in every class. Ceiling fans or central air conditioning are a must. The floor must be wood finished or a smooth tile, as students dance barefoot. The room must have no obstructions in order to enable students to move freely.

The Teacher's Role

In Western culture, the teacher is the leader of the class and everyone takes their lead from her, even the drummer. The teacher dictates the mood of the class by studying her students and knows how fast or slow to move the class overall. The teacher sticks to her syllabus for the semester. The teacher first performs each dance so students can see exactly what the dance looks like before they learn it. The teacher gives a 15–20-minute lecture on the background and history of the dance before teaching it to the students so they understand the dance.

Attention in Class

Attention is given to each and every student in class. Some students may not need much attention, while others may need quite a bit. The instructor will study every student in class first by their African name characteristic, which gives an idea what they are and how to handle each one. The buddy system mentioned earlier allows students to practice with each other and in as many groups as possible. You will also be encouraged to reach out to the instructor if you need extra help with the dances. These specifics will be elaborated further in Chapter 2.

Learning about the Dance Form: History, Artists, Major Works, Styles, and Aesthetics

The students have to pay close attention to the teacher, drummer, and dance instruction in order to implement the steps. There is no counting in African dancing, so listening to the rhythms of the drums is very important in order to keep to the downbeat. It can be easy, yet can also be challenging, but this book will see you through.

At George Mason University, the history behind the dance is taught, and the African artists are introduced, including their genre of music, their styles and aesthetics, and all their major works. This takes the student on a journey to Africa without a passport.

Student Etiquette

Mentally, the students should prepare to comprehend what they are about to undertake which can be absolutely foreign to their bodies the very first time. No gum chewing in class; no cell phones allowed; courtesy to peers is emphasized; respect to the teacher is required; gratitude to the drummer is expected; and proper attire is a must.

African dance is done in bare feet so one can feel the connection to Mother Earth (this is all explained in detail in Chapter 2). Stamina is built in this class, as the students learn all 10 dances by the end of the semester. The African dos and don'ts are explained at the beginning of taking this class, which helps the students understand the importance of etiquette in Africa.

This book will prepare you for your first time as an African dance class student. You will know how to dress for class, behave in class, and what to expect in class. You will practice courtesy, respect, endurance, effort, perseverance, and discipline in class. African dance is more than just dance; it's a discipline in life.

At George Mason University, attendance goes toward the student's grade, and this is made known to the student right at the beginning of the class. If a student is late for class, they must sit out and take notes and cannot dance that day. This encourages the students to attend class on time. Generally, this isn't an issue since the class is so important to most students that they hate to miss class or be late because they know they will miss the beginning of story time.

However, if you must enter class after it is in session, you must pay your respects by entering quietly and sitting on the side until you are permitted to join the class. You may not be permitted to join the class, depending on how late you are. If you need to leave early for any given reason, you will need to inform the teacher before the start of the class via e-mail or another manner. Students are allowed a necessary water and bathroom break in between dance sessions as a class, as opposed to individually, to avoid excuses.

Safety First

For safety and flexibility, every student, regardless of gender, must change from street clothes to dance workout clothes or sportswear for class. Because African dance is traditionally taught and performed barefoot and to prevent damaging the studio floor, you must remove your shoes as soon as you get to the studio. To prevent cramping and illness, you have to eat two hours before the class, or else eat after class is over. For safety, anyone with long hair must tie their hair up in a bun or otherwise ensure that it stays out of their face and other students' faces. With the repetition of head and neck movements, long hair left loose will impair your view and diminish the enjoyment. These specifics will be elaborated on in Chapters 2 and 3.

Course Requirements

Course requirements are individual and specified by individual professors and universities. For classes at George Mason University, every student is expected to know all ten dances and is required to choose three out of the ten to practice and perfect for their finals. Students need to know the background and story for any dance they choose. They are required to prepare each dance to be performed as a solo in front of the rest of the class for grading. Students are also required to do a double-spaced paper on each dance and will be graded on their papers, as well as their solo performances.

The following are the requirements expected of the students in African Dance Class at GMU:

- Attendance and participation: 20%
- Growth, development, progress: 10%
- Technical ability: 10%
- Written work: 10%
- Concert attendance: 10%
- Final movement exam: 40%

Attending Dance Class

At George Mason University, each student is required to attend all 14 or 15 weeks of class within the given semester. African dance class is offered twice a week, and attendance is about ten percent of the student's final grade. Students are allowed to be absent a maximum of three times in the semester and will have to catch up on missed classes from the buddy system created at the beginning of the semester. The importance of attendance is seen in the performance of the student.

If a student misses class, first of all, she misses the story time of the dance, which explains the background of the dance and its in-depth details. Secondly, she misses the firsthand breakdown of the dances taught by the instructor. Lastly, she misses the actual repetition of the dance that is so much needed to perfect the dance. These three factors are important in the learning of a dance—that it pushes the students to attend class. Instructors will make the classes so much fun by having the students practice in small and large groups, and at times in two large groups against each other, making them alert to the movements and giving them a competitive attitude, which physiologically makes them want to be better at the dances in front of their peers.

Performing Dance Combinations

African dance is taught in segments of body isolations. It is a dance that has to be broken down for you to learn the combinations. It demands the movement of about five components of your body at one time. This book will enable you to learn and break down the steps so that you will be able to accomplish the African dances.

Analyzing Movement and Steps

Students are encouraged to take notes during class and to watch attentively to the movements and steps to each dance taught so they can prepare to take the dance class. During the dance class sessions, the teacher takes a few minutes to explain each movement and step so the students may know exactly what the dance entails and how to properly execute it.

Attending Performances

Students are required to attend the university's dance company concerts. This introduces various dance techniques to the students on an entertainment basis. The dance school encourages this type of activity as part of the class curriculum, so every student is expected to attend two mandatory school performances. Students are required to turn in their ticket stubs and programs so the professor can add that as an extra credit toward their final grades. Other extra curriculum performances are also encouraged in my African dance class to enable the students to attend other African dances outside of the school so they can be exposed to the different cultures of Africa.

THE CONTINENT OF AFRICA

Countries, Capitals, and Languages

Of the 56 countries and regions in the continent of Africa, there are only six that speak Portuguese: Angola, Mozambique, São Tomé and Principe, Cape Verde, Guinea-Bissau, and Equatorial Guinea. There only two that speak Spanish: Equatorial Guinea and Western Sahara. Djibouti is the only country that has the same name as its capital. The highest mountain in Africa is Mt. Kilimanjaro. The two main deserts in Africa are the Sahara Desert and the Kalahari Desert. The two longest rivers in Africa are the Nile River and the Congo River. The two largest lakes in Africa are Lake Victoria and Lake Tanganyika.

Overview of African Village Life

African villages vary across regions of the continent. To understand the hierarchy and social stratification, the **Akan** people of Ghana, West Africa, will be discussed. Villages are made up of people within the same tribe who speak the same language. Within a tribe are various clans, with specific family crests that describe the clan. This author, for instance, is of the *twidan* clan of the Fante-speaking tribe, which is under the Akan group. There is a Fante king, or **hene**, for a region, but also chiefs who govern specific villages and their council of elders, who help them rule. A **queen mother** is also an important part of Akan royalty, a title reserved for senior women in the royal matrilineage. Within a clan are family elders who oversee matters ranging from birth to death.

Milestones are celebrated by families within a clan with invitations extended to friends. **Amambra**, or traditions, have been practiced for centuries. Music and dance are an integral part of celebrations in African villages. It is common during festivals to see whole communities dancing in the streets, so to speak. Most celebrations culminate in dance. Whether a child is being named at an outdoor ceremony or a family member is buried, each of these opposing celebrations results in dancing.

African Dance in Community Settings

African dance is a shared activity within the communities in Africa. Gatherings are very common, which start up celebrations involving dancing. For example, a typical community gathering happens under a real big old tree that has produced so many branches that give extended shading. The people of a tribe come out from their homes and sit under this tree to enjoy food and drink brought by various families for sharing. The drummers from all over the communities come with their drums (like a drum circle), and drumbeats begin to sound out loud.

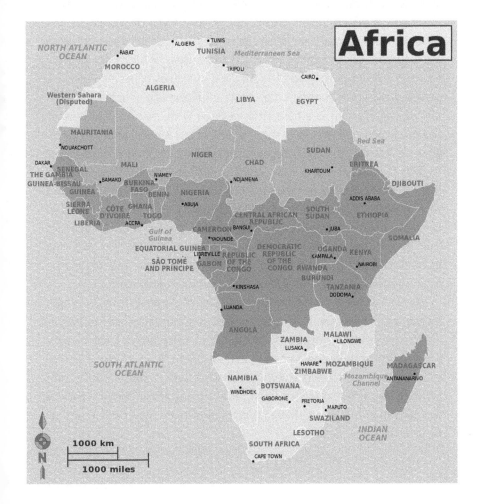

Figure 1.1 Map of Africa

Then, dancers in the communities also come out and in response to the drums begin to dance. Depending on the tribe or region, origins of drumbeats are recognized by their beats and rhythms. A dancer can differentiate between the beats of the drums and know which dances to perform. As previously mentioned, dancing for Africans starts very early at the age of three, so the experience is acquired very early.

Values of Dance in Africa

The values of African dance are vast in number. They are an important aspect of the African life, as well as being the basis for unification. Throughout the continent, dance is used as a form of recreation and entertainment among the tribes; it teaches social patterns and values to the members of the community. Rural tribal areas of Africa do not have a strong written history, so the traditions and rules of each society are passed down from generation to generation through dance, music, and storytelling. Dancing is a custom associated with important gatherings and milestones in the lives of the villagers, so it is viewed as an opportunity to come together as a community and share a common connection.

The flexibility of the limbs used in African dances also prepares one for the flexibility of other genres of dance. It frees the spirit and allows one to express their joyful feelings outwardly while engaged in the dances. One can see deep smiles on all the faces of the dancers and the expressions they exude, along with cheerful laughs that ring through the dancing. The dance calls that come from the lips of the dancers are heard far and wide as they perform their dances.

As you venture further into the realm of African dance, you will realize it is more than body isolations. It will introduce you to movements you never thought possible, but it will also provide the history and culture of the people of this vast continent. You will gain a better appreciation for the complexities of traditions, tribes, culture, and heritage. You will realize that music and dancing are an integral part of the African culture, and that modern-day dances owe their roots to African dances.

Tribes of the Continent of Africa

There are many different ethnic groups and tribes across the continent of Africa, with their culture varying from tribe to tribe. In order for you to become familiar with the tribes of Africa, below is a representative list of some of the tribes and their countries of origin.

Afar

The Afar people live primarily in Ethiopia and the areas of Eritrea, Djibouti, and Somalia in the Horn of Africa.

Akan

The Akan are the largest ethnic group in Ghana and the Ivory Coast. They are broken into many subgroups, including the Asante, Fante and Wassa. Their culture is traditionally matrilineal.

Amhara

The Amhara are the politically and culturally dominant ethnic group of Ethiopia. They are located primarily in the central highland plateau of Ethiopia and comprise the major population element in the provinces of Begemder and Gojjam and in parts of Shoa and Wallo.

Anlo-Ewe

The Anlo-Ewe people are today in the southeastern corner of the Republic of Ghana. They settled here around 1474 after escaping from their past home of Notsie.

Ashanti

The Ashanti live in central Ghana in western Africa, approximately 300 km. away from the coast. The Ashanti are a major ethnic group of the Akans in Ghana, a fairly new nation, barely more than 50 years old.

Bakongo

The Bakongo people (also called the Kongo) dwell along the Atlantic coast of Africa from Pointe-Noire, Congo (Brazzaville), to Luanda, Angola.

Bambara

The Bambara are a large Mande racial group located mostly in the country of Mali. They are the largest and most dominant group in that country.

Bemba

The Bemba are located in the northeastern part of Zambia and are the largest ethnic group in the northern province of Zambia.

Berber

Berbers have lived in Africa since earliest recorded time. References date back to 3000 B.C. There are many scattered tribes of Berber across Morocco, Algeria, Tunisia, Libya, and Egypt.

Bobo

The Bobo people have lived in western Burkina Faso and Mali for centuries. They are known for their masks, which are worn with elaborate outfits for celebrations. Primarily agricultural people, they also cultivate cotton, which they use to trade with others.

Bushmen/San

The "Bushmen" are the oldest inhabitants of southern Africa, where they have lived for at least 20,000 years. Their home is in the vast expanse of the Kalahari Desert.

Chewa

The Chewa, also known as the Cewa or Chichewa, is an African culture that has existed since the beginning of the first millennium A.D. They are primarily located in Zambia, Zimbabwe, with the bulk of the population in Malawi.

Dogon

The Dogon are a cliff-dwelling people who live in southeastern Mali and Burkina Faso. Among the people groups in Africa, they are unique in that they have kept and continued to develop their own culture, even in the midst of Islamic invasions. These invasions conquered and adapted many of the current people groups.

Fang

The Fang are especially known for their guardian figures, which they attach to wooden boxes containing the bones of ancestors. The bones, by tradition, are said to contain the power of the dead person—in fact, the same amount of power that the person had while still alive.

Fon

The Fon of Benin (originally called Dahomey until 1975) are from West Africa. The Fon are said to have originated in the area of Tado, a town in Togo, at approximately the same latitude as Abomey, Benin.

Fulani

The Fulani people of West Africa are the largest nomadic group in the world, primarily nomadic herders and traders. Through their nomadic lifestyle, they established numerous trade routes in West Africa.

Ibos

From Nigeria, the Ibos live in villages that have anywhere from a few hundred to a few thousand people comprised of numerous extended families.

Kikuyu (Gikuyu)

Having migrated to their current location about four centuries ago, the Kikuyu now make up Kenya's largest ethnic group.

Maasai

The Maasai, famous as herders and warriors, once dominated the plains of East Africa. Now, however, they are confined to a fraction of their former range.

Mandinka

The Mandinka are an ethnic group living in West Africa, mostly in Senegal, Gambia, and Guinea-Bissau, but some also live in Burkina Faso, Mali, and Côte d'Ivoire.

Pygmies

There are many different "Pygmy" peoples—for example, the Bambuti, the Batwa, the Bayaka, and the Bagyeli (*Ba-* means people)—who live scattered over a huge area in central and western Africa, in the Democratic Republic of Congo (DRC), Congo (Brazzaville), Cameroon, Gabon, Central African Republic, Rwanda, Burundi, and Uganda.

Samburu

The Samburu are related to the Maasai, although they live just above the equator, where the foothills of Mt. Kenya merge into the northern desert and slightly south of Lake Turkana in the Rift Valley Province of Kenya.

Senufo

The Senufo are a group of people living in northern Côte d'Ivoire and Mali. They are known as excellent farmers and are made up of a number of different groups who moved south to Mali and Côte d'Ivoire in the 15th and 16th centuries.

Tuareg

The Tuareg people are predominantly nomadic people of the Sahara desert, mostly in the northern reaches of Mali, near Timbuktu and Kidal.

Wolof

The Wolof are one of the largest groups to inhabit modern-day Senegal. They live anywhere from the desert area of the Sahara to the rain forests. Traditionally, many Wolof lived in small villages governed by an extended family unit, but now most Wolof move to cities where they are able to get jobs.

Yoruba

The Yoruba people live in southwest Nigeria and Benin. They have developed a variety of different artistic forms, including pottery, weaving, beadwork, metalwork, and mask making.

Zulu

The Zulu are the largest ethnic group in South Africa. They are well known for their beautiful brightly colored beads and baskets, as well as other small carvings.

Symbolic Meanings of Color in Africa[1]

YELLOW in all its variations is associated with the yolk of the egg, ripe and edible fruits and vegetables, and also with the mineral gold. In some spiritual purification rituals, mashed yam is rendered yellow with oil palm and served with eggs. It symbolizes sanctity, preciousness, royalty, wealth, spirituality, vitality, and fertility.

PINK is associated with the female essence of life. It is viewed as red rendered mild and gentle, and therefore associated with tenderness, calmness, pleasantness, and sweetness. According to Akan social thought, these attributes are generally considered as core aspects of the female essence.

RED is associated with blood, sacrificial rites, and the shedding of blood. Red-eyed mood means a sense of seriousness, readiness for a serious spiritual or political encounter. Red is therefore used as a symbol of heightened spiritual and political mood, sacrifice, and struggle.

BLUE is associated with the blue sky, the abode of the Supreme Creator. It is thus used in a variety of ways to symbolize spiritual sanctity, good fortune, peacefulness, harmony, and love-related ideas.

GREEN is associated with vegetation, planting, harvesting, and herbal medicine. Tender green leaves are usually used to sprinkle water during purification rituals. It symbolizes growth, vitality, fertility, prosperity, fruitfulness, abundant health, and spiritual rejuvenation.

PURPLE is viewed in the same way as maroon. It is considered as earth associated with color used in rituals and healing purposes. This

---

1   Ofori-Ansa, 2009

color is also used in rituals and healing purposes. It is also associated with feminine aspects of life. Females mostly wear purple clothes.

MAROON has a close resemblance to red-brown, which is associated with the color of Mother Earth. Red-brown is usually obtained from clay and is therefore associated with healing and the power to repel malevolent spirits.

WHITE derives its symbolism from the white part of the egg and from white clay used in spiritual purification, healing, sanctification rites, and festive occasions. In some situations, it symbolizes contact with ancestral spirits, deities, and other unknown spiritual entities such as ghosts. It is used in combination with black, green, or yellow to express motion, spirituality, vitality, and balance.

GRAY derives its symbolism from ash. Ash is used for healing and spiritual cleansing rituals to recreate spiritual balance when spiritual blemish has occurred. It is also used in rituals for protection against malevolent spirits. Grey is thus associated with spiritual blemish, but also with spiritual cleansing.

SILVER is associated with the moon, which represents the female essence of life. Silver ornaments are usually worn by women and are used in the context of spiritual purification, naming ceremonies, marriage ceremonies, and other community festivals. It symbolizes serenity, purity, and joy.

GOLD derives its significance from the commercial value and social prestige associated with the precious mineral. Gold dust and gold nuggets were used as mediums of exchange and for making valuable royal ornaments. It symbolizes royalty, wealth, elegance, high status, supreme quality, glory, and spiritual purity.

BLACK derives its significance from the notion that new things get darker as they mature; physical aging comes with spiritual maturity. The Akans blacken most of their ritual objects to increase their spiritual potency. Black symbolizes an intensified spiritual energy, communion with the ancestral spirits, antiquity, spiritual maturity, and spiritual potency. Colors are chosen for both their visual effect and their symbolic meanings.

African Soul Names and Characteristics (from the Fante tribe)[2]

The following are the male and female soul names of the week in the Akan tribe of Ghana.

A name represents the very being of a person. Every name has a meaning, character, and history. An African child is forever reminded by his given name of who she is and who she represents.

	MALES	PRONOUNCED	FEMALES	PRONOUNCED
Monday:	Kodwo	ko-jo	Adwowa	aa-ju-wa
Tuesday:	Kobina	ko-be-na	Araba	aa-ra-ba
Wednesday:	Kweku	quee-ku	Ekua	ay-ku-wa
Thursday:	Yaw	ya-wo	Aba	aa-b-a
Friday:	Kofi	ko-fee	Efua	ay-fu-wa
Saturday:	Kwame	qu-waa-me	Ama	aa-ma
Sunday:	Kwesi	quee-cee	Esi	ay-cee

Characteristics of the African Soul Names

In Western culture, some people believe in horoscopes that tell you what zodiac sign you are. In the Akan culture of the people of Ghana, they believe in the days of the week depicting the characteristics of the day the child was born. These characteristics are so true to point and have been passed down from generation to generation. At the beginning of every semester, the instructor gives the students homework to find their African Soul Names from handouts from class. Students put in their date of birth along with the year they were born, and this gives them the exact day of the week they were born. Students have to hold onto this name throughout the semester as the instructor calls out attendance by their Soul names. Most students keep their African Soul names even after they have graduated from African dance class. They find this amazing and enjoy the fact that they have an African Soul Name.

---

2   Kyereboah, 2006

Monday Child: Father or mother of the family, a nurturer, dependable and organized, and protective of his family.

Tuesday Child: The planner of the family, structured in nature, neutral in all matters, never taking sides, problem solver.

Wednesday Child: Fully in control of every situation, does not want to be told what to do, knows it all, spontaneous, vibrant, and cordial, but do not cross her path.

Thursday Child: Quiet in nature, very observant, taking it all in, a listener, not a talker, but analyzes every situation very well.

Friday Child: A leader, not a follower, very temperamental, but has a big heart, always the instigator of everything.

Saturday Child: Likes to take control of family situations. Running the show and making the rules, but will go out of her way for others anytime.

Sunday Child: Passive, sensitive, warm, and tends to be shy, likes to keep to himself, but very aware of his surroundings and usually the secret keeper of the family.

Regions/African Countries (56)

REGION	COUNTRY	CAPITAL	LANGUAGES
CENTRAL (9)			
CENTRAL	Angola	Luanda	Portuguese
CENTRAL	Cameroon	Yaounde	French, English
CENTRAL	Central African Republic	Bangui	Arabic, French
CENTRAL	Chad	N'Djamena	French, Arabic
CENTRAL	Congo	Brazzaville	French
CENTRAL	Democratic Rep. of the Congo	Kinshasa	French
CENTRAL	Equatorial Guinea	Malabo	Spanish, French, Portuguese
CENTRAL	Gabon	Libreville	French
CENTRAL	São Tomé & Principe	São Tomé	French, Portuguese
EAST (17)			
EAST	Burundi	Bujumbura	French
EAST	Comoros	Moroni	French, Arabic
EAST	Djibouti	Djibouti	French, Arabic

EAST	Eritrea	Asmara	English, Arabic
EAST	Ethiopia	Addis Ababa	English
EAST	Kenya	Nairobi	English
EAST	Madagascar	Antananarivo	French
EAST	Malawi	Lilongwe	English
EAST	Mauritius	Port Louis	English, French
EAST	Mozambique	Maputo	Portuguese
EAST	Rwanda	Kigali	French, English
EAST	Seychelles	Victoria	French, English
EAST	Somalia	Mogadishu	English, Arabic, Italian
EAST	Somaliland	Hargeisa	English, Arabic
EAST	Tanzania	Dodoma/Dar Es Salaam	English
EAST	Uganda	Kampala	English
EAST	Zambia	Lusaka	English
NORTH (8)			
NORTH	Algeria	Algiers	French, Arabic
NORTH	Egypt	Cairo	English, Arabic
NORTH	Libya	Tripoli	English, Arabic, Italian
NORTH	Morocco	Rabat	Arabic, French
NORTH	South Sudan	Juba	English
NORTH	Republic of Sudan	Khartoum	English, Arabic
NORTH	Tunisia	Tunis	French, Arabic
NORTH	Western Sahara	El Aaiun	Spanish, Arabic
SOUTH (6)			
SOUTH	Botswana	Gaborone	English
SOUTH	Lesotho	Maseru	English
SOUTH	Namibia	Windhoek	English
SOUTH	South Africa	Pretoria/Cape Town	English
SOUTH	Swaziland	Mbabane	English
SOUTH	Zimbabwe	Harare	English
WEST (16)			
WEST	Benin	Porto-Novo/ Cotonou	French
WEST	Burkina Faso	Ouagadougou	French
WEST	Cape Verde	Praia	Portuguese

WEST	Gambia	Banjul	English
WEST	Ghana	Accra	English
WEST	Guinea-Bissau	Bissau	Portuguese
WEST	Guinea	Conakry	French
WEST	Ivory Coast	Abidjan/ Yamoussoukro	French
WEST	Liberia	Monrovia	English
WEST	Mali	Bamako	French
WEST	Mauritania	Nouakchott	Arabic, French
WEST	Niger	Niamey	French, Arabic
WEST	Nigeria	Abuja	English
WEST	Senegal	Dakar	French
WEST	Sierra Leone	Freetown	English
WEST	Togo	Lome	French

GLOSSARY

Akan	An ethnic group predominantly in Ghana, West Africa
Amambra	An Akan word that means traditions
Boombsey	A jovial term relating to the buttocks
Hene	An Akan word for king
Outdooring	A naming ceremony for an Akan infant
Polyrhythm	The simultaneous use of two or more conflicting rhythms that are not readily perceived as deriving from one another, or as simple manifestations of the same meter (Wikipedia)
Queen Mother	Female royalty whose power is matrilineal
Story Time	A period at the beginning of dance class used to introduce the history behind the dance

REFERENCES

Kyereboah, N. (2006). *Soul Name*. Midlothian, VA: Nabina Publications.

Locke, D. (1998). *Drum Gahu*. Gilsum, NH: White Cliffs Media.

Nettleford, R. (1996). *African Dance*. Africa World Press, Inc.

Ofori-Ansa, K. (2009). *Ashanti Kente Cloth—More than a Piece of Fabric: A Part of Culture*. Retrieved January 2013 from http://kente.midwesttradegroup .com/history.html

Welsh, K. (2004). *African Dance*. Philadelphia: Chelsea House Publishers, 2004.

Welsh Asante, K. (2000). *Zimbabwe Dance*. Trenton, NJ: Africa World Press, Inc.

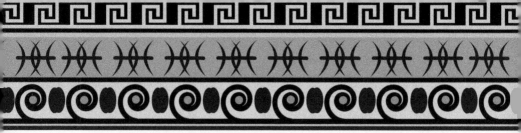

Chapter 2

MIND-BODY PREPARATION FOR DANCE CLASS

A frican dance is a state of mind which requires the body, mind, and soul to be synchronized. Whether the quest of the student is to tone their body, learn African dance for enjoyment or knowledge, or just to experience a spiritually liberating set of movements, this genre will deliver those results.

Before attending dance class, you should be aware of the way you will need to dress. There are criteria for the way to dress that will allow you to mimic the dance movements. African dance protocols and class structure are unlike any other dance class of Western influence you may have experienced. The protocols and class structure that you will follow will transport you right in the midst of selected African cultures. In addition to being cognizant of the attire and protocols, you will have to be mentally and physically prepared in order to reap the benefits of this class.

AFRICAN DANCE PREPARATION CHECKLIST

1. Wear clothes that allow you to move with no resistance.
2. Be prepared to dance barefoot or wear a foot thong.
3. Long hair should be tied in a bun.

29

4. Eat at least two hours before class.
5. Bring a towel and water bottle.
6. Prepare mentally and physically for a cultural journey.
7. No street clothes, electronics, or gum allowed.
8. Expect to burn 800 to 1000 calories per class.
9. Small muscle groups will be used and felt.
10. Be prepared to be part of a community and have fun!

DRESSING FOR CLASS

When enrolling in an African dance class, you should be aware of the clothing that is expected for class. You will not be able to attend class in street clothes such as jeans, dress pants, dress shorts, dress shirts, and blouses. Be prepared to be clothed in the specified attire that is recommended. Imagine showing up to ballet class dressed in sweats. The pirouette or plié would not be comfortable, and the fluidity of dance may be interrupted. The same is true for African dance. The clothing is, therefore, an important part of the preparation.

Students taking African dance should wear clothes that allow them to move with no resistance. Each part of the body moves and extends to the beats of drums. Restrictive clothing will not allow the students to fully extend and appreciate the choreography. Students should choose clothing such as exercise pants, yoga pants, gym shorts, T-shirts, and leotards. All women should wear sports bras for aerobics, and women with well-endowed bosoms may opt to wear two aerobics sports bras for better support. Any dangling or loose jewelry needs to be removed prior to dance class.

DANCING BAREFOOT

African dance is performed barefoot. The main reason for barefoot dancing is so that the dancer can connect to Mother Earth, as she is referred to in African cultures. The soles of the dancer's feet respond to the beats of the drums that resonate underground right through the feet. Shoes or sneakers would not allow the dancer to properly translate the beats to movement, and it would not be authentic. If dancing barefoot is challenging for you, **foot thongs** may be worn. Foot thongs are slip-on, partial foot coverings that cover the ball of the foot. Depending on the manufacturer, foot thongs are sometimes called Dance Paws or Foot Undeez.

AFRICAN DANCE CLASS STRUCTURE

Protocol

In African cultures, protocol is an integral part of normal routines. The same is true for the dance class, which is a microcosm of the African cultures whose dances are being learned. The structure of the class is designed to allow you to experience the totality of African dance. In addition to the etiquette described in the first chapter, other rules may be implemented as the need arises to address any distractions.

Class Structure

Each African dance has its own story. At George Mason University, the story is told to the students as a "story time" before performing. The teacher explains the genre of dance, the story behind the dance, and the meaning of the dance.

Students then form two rows facing the instructor and drummer. The shorter students are in the front row and the taller students are in the back row. Depending on the size of the studio, the rows may include as many as ten students apiece. After the rows have been formed, each student spreads out their arms and turns 360 degrees to establish their personal space. The space between each student should be ample enough that their hands do not touch. This beginning formation allows the instructor to walk among the rows and individually observe students. When the instructor notices incorrect execution of the dance, you receive immediate one-on-one feedback, regardless of the class size. This configuration is known as the **African dance practice line**. The first person in the line is the leader because he is the closest to the instructor. A variation of the line formation is students moving in a circle from the front of the class to the back of the class. As they dance, the instructor stands in front of the class and is able to notice each student as they circle to the front.

The Role of a Live Drummer

The drummer and his beats synchronize the dance instruction. In African dance, one must follow the beat of the drums in movement and start moving on the downbeat, as counting is not a common practice for dancing in African society. For every new dance movement, the drummer first plays at a slow tempo, then increases his accompaniment to a medium tempo, and finally a faster tempo when he observes students can perform the movements at each tempo.

Welsh, quoting Opoku, wrote, "Drumming, singing, and clapping play an equally important 'role in the drama of African community life. They set the scene, create the mood and the atmosphere' for the dancer to interpret music through symbolic gestures, bodily movements, and facial expressions."

Dance Structure

A **dance movement** entails one particular form of physical expression that uses one or more body parts to tell a story. However, a **movement sequence** involves a combination of two dance movements. Within a class period, several movement sequences are taught. A dance performance includes three to five movement sequences. For example, the dance **Djolo** has five complete movement sequences altogether.

The beginning of every dance movement has its protocol as well. Each movement must begin on the right side because the right hand is considered the respectful hand. Starting on the left hand is disrespectful. This is customary growing up in **Ghana**. Whenever a child greets an adult, she is expected to shake with her right hand, even if she is left handed. It is corrected if a child offers her left hand to an adult. The same goes for handing an object to an adult with the left hand; it will not be received unless the object is placed in the right hand and given to the adult.

In African dance, opposite movements are considered a complete movement sequence. When you move forward and backward, you have completed one movement sequence. Likewise, when you move to the right and left or clockwise and counterclockwise, or up and down, those pairs all constitute one movement sequence. In essence, a dance step consisting of four movement sequences actually has eight dance movements to the sequence.

You will be required to keep your eyes on the instructor at all times while dancing. African dance will be taught in movement sequences. At the conclusion of the instruction, the class will return in rows to their original positions to perform. The whole dance is performed eight times, and the tall students then switch with the short students in the front and repeat the process. Students may also be separated into five or six groups so that they can be monitored closely and their techniques honed.

You can expect to learn ten dances in a semester and will choose two or three of them to perfect and perform for finals.

Group Practice

In addition to individual practices, the class will be divided into smaller groups to perform the dances. Groups on either side of the class will switch positions and continue to practice. This process continues until the class has practiced the routine eight times. This section of class is termed the dance marathon. Within an hour class, 45 minutes of it is spent practicing.

At the beginning of the semester, each student is paired up to another called a "buddy," who practices with you outside of class. Sometimes, you will be paired with your buddy in class and encouraged to discuss and practice the dances being taught. After approximately five minutes, pairs are randomly called to perform for the class. In this configuration, the majority of the class is seated on one side of the room as the audience and the pairs or small groups perform on the opposite side of the room—the stage. The audience is encouraged to give praise as well as constructive criticism. This exercise allows for you to further grow in your dancing and prepares you for your final performance examinations. It also strips you of any shyness you may have overall. Students appear to thoroughly enjoy this format.

Practice is not confined to the classroom. You are encouraged to practice with your buddy in and out of class. The buddy does not have to be the same gender. In the event you miss class, your buddy will teach you the steps, bringing you up to speed with the class upon your return. You should be aware that you, the dancer, are an independent performer and solely responsible for your final performance.

Ending Class

The class always starts facing the drummer and instructor and ends in that same fashion. At the conclusion of class, the drummer is thanked in a unique fashion. You and the entire class will get down on your knees and drum on the floor as you are accompanied by the drummer's beats. Students only cease their drumming when the drummer stops. This gesture is considered the highest form of gratitude to the drummer.

Just as the drummer is given his merit, the instructor is also thanked in a unique way. After the class, the students will position themselves facing the instructor with their left hand behind them, and then the right hand beats against the chest twice, slides forward from the chin, and extends out toward the instructor. With the proper thanks given, the class can be dismissed.

At the end of class, students sit in a circle and take deep breaths to calm themselves for their next class. You will be asked to verbally share your thoughts on the class, as well as evaluate the dance steps. This allows you to express whatever unresolved questions you might have prior to leaving class.

The day after class, you may be slightly sore in common muscular areas as you would expect, but you may also be sore in smaller muscle groups. Core muscles are utilized extensively in the African dance class. You may be pleasantly surprised that dance movements learned in class can be taken to the dance floor.

Students have expressed that the protocols, rules, and discipline of the African dance class help direct them toward a structured environment which serves more than one purpose. On one hand, it allows you to master the dances taught, but on the other hand, this structure is far reaching and contributes to the molding of other areas in your life.

PREPARING PHYSICALLY AND MENTALLY FOR CLASS

You should prepare for the authenticity of the class. Any precon-ceived notions of what African dance should be, as defined by others, should be discarded. A famous pop star was filming her video and wanted the choreography to include African dance. She enlisted the help of several African American dance groups, or so she thought. As she watched each group perform, she found herself thinking something was missing, and the dance movements did not feel or look authentic. It appeared the movements she was observing were Westernized. Disappointed with what she was seeing, she decided to track down three young African men she had seen online to dance for her in person. When they danced, she knew they were just what she needed for her video. Their moves, in her opinion, appeared to come from within and not taught. She worked hard with them until she perfected their moves, as well as included them in her video.

Preparing for class both physically and mentally is important. There is an old Fante **proverb** (Fante is a dialect of Ghana, West Africa) that states *Ohia nyansa na ahow ɔdzin a ma abaawa etum e twa no ho asaw.* Translated in English, it means: "It requires strength and wisdom for a young lady to dance."

Physical Preparation

Physically, you should stretch and warm up your muscles before move-ment begins. As with any form of activity, inadequate warm-ups prior to the activity may cause injury. Food should be consumed at least two hours before class to allow adequate digestion. Failure to allow this time lapse may result in vomiting. A bottle of water and a towel is recom-mended, as African dancing is very vibrant and energetic. You do not have to be in shape prior to taking the class. Learning African dances increases your endurance. Breathing through the nose and out through the mouth is a breathing technique that you will learn to help you endure.

The student should gain a heightened **kinesthetic** sense. Kinesthesia is the sense that detects bodily position, weight, or movement of muscles, tendons, and joints. In African dance, four or five different components of your body are moved at a time, and this utilizes both small and large muscle groups. This is in contrast to Western dances, in which the head and neck are not moved as much.

You should plan for your body to experience certain physical aspects after the first class. You should expect to be slightly tired, but continue exercising in order to build stamina. In class, you should expect to burn between 800 to 1000 calories per class. This may result in being drenched in sweat after class. You should plan to shower following this activity. Added bonuses expressed by students are the weight loss and exhilaration the class provides.

Mental Preparation

You should prepare mentally to comprehend what you are about to experience. African dance movements are different from how you are accustomed to moving. This may be foreign to your body and may feel awkward until you have mastered it. You need to be mentally prepared for a vigorous routine. For some, it might be more vigorous than hip hop or ballet. All components of the body are engaged from head to toe. If you exercise outside of class, you will reap the benefits in increased endurance. You should focus on learning the dance steps on your own and refrain from observing your neighbor.

The African dance reaches beyond movement and teaches life lessons. A student e-mailed that the class was too difficult, and she was quitting. She was told that if she quits this, she would quit anything that comes along in her life that was challenging. Although she did not entirely agree, at the time, she stayed with the dance and became one of the best students. She later stated that the advice changed her life.

You are ready to take an African dance class. Before you do, review the preparations to help you get the best out of the class. First, being dressed appropriately is important to be able to learn the dance moves. Next, be prepared for the protocol that exists, some of which is an extension of the cultures whose dances you will be learning. Finally, you must be physically and mentally prepared.

GLOSSARY

African dance practice line	Two lines of students facing the instructor with a gap between for the instructor to stroll and observe
Core muscles	Muscles that help stabilize and move the pelvis and spine
Dance movement	A physical expression that uses one or more body parts
Djolo	An African female initiation dance
Fante	An Akan dialect spoken in Ghana, West Africa
Foot thong	Slip-on, partial foot coverings that cover the ball of the foot
Ghana	An African country on the west coast of the continent, previously known as the Gold Coast
Kinesthetic	The kinesthetic sense detects bodily position, weight, or movement of muscles, tendons, and joints
Movement sequence	Two or more dance movements
Proverb	A simple and popular saying that expresses a basic truth

REFERENCE

Welsh, K. (with quote by Alfred Mawere Opoku). (2004). *African Dance*. Philadelphia: Chelsea House Publishers.

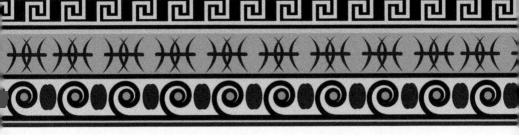

Chapter 3

HEALTH AND SAFETY ATTRIBUTES OF DANCE

S afe African dance classes should always have a warm-up segment in the beginning and a cooldown segment at the end to prevent risk of injury and allow gradual heart rate increase and decrease. Safety and injury prevention are important aspects in African dance. The conditions of the studio are also important in contributing to an optimum experience.

STUDIO SAFETY

The studio should have adequate ventilation for proper breathing. The temperature should be around 70°F to accommodate the elevated body temperature when the students are dancing. The floors of the studio should be constructed of wood, linoleum, or vinyl dance floor material and be devoid of any imperfections. These items are particularly important because students will be dancing barefoot. Only water bottles should be used, and students should be mindful of cleaning up any spilled water immediately. Students should not lean on mirrors. Include the steps students should take to make sure that the studio is safe for dance classes. Finally, there should be adequate spacing above the head to allow for each student to reach up without touching the ceiling.

PERSONAL SAFETY

As mentioned in Chapter 2, you should wear appropriate loose clothing and secure long hair. If you are not able to dance barefoot, foot thongs may be used to protect the balls of the feet. You will need to control your breathing to help pace you throughout the class, due to the energetic movements that can make you tired and exhausted. Prior to dancing, you must answer the following questions about your health. If the answer is yes to any of the questions, you need to seek a physician's advice and clearance:

- Do you have any respiratory problems such as asthma, chronic bronchitis, emphysema, or any shortness of breath during exercise?
- Do you have sudden bursts of rapid heartbeats or any heart troubles?
- Do you have any pain or sensation of pressure in your chest when participating in any form of exercise?
- Does your heart ever beat unevenly, irregularly, or skip beats?
- Do you take any prescription medicine on a regular basis?
- Do you have any blood pressure problems?
- Have you had any dizzy spells, or do you often feel faint during exercise?
- Do you have a bone or joint problem such as arthritis that gets worse with dancing?
- Do you have any back or knee problems that will prohibit you from dancing?
- Do you have any physical condition that you need to divulge to your dance instructor before you participate in class?

In addition, if you are injured, you will need a doctor's note for class and will be relegated to taking observation notes. It is essential that injured students refrain from dancing, as this might cause further injury to the body.

BASIC DANCE ANATOMY AND KINESIOLOGY

As a student of African dance, expect to learn the basic knowledge of dance anatomy and **kinesiology**, which will give you a better understanding of the body movements. Kinesiology is the study of human movement. African dance is cardiovascular in nature, which means the movements require sustained activity that trains the heart, lungs, and muscles to use oxygen directly for energy. All the movements are low impact, but require high energy, which is aerobic energy production. **Aerobic** means exercises that require oxygen such as:

- Dance fitness
- Running
- Jogging
- Walking
- Biking

On the contrary, **anaerobic** exercise means without oxygen. These are stop-and-go activities like weight lifting.

Anatomy

During dance, the muscles receive oxygen from the bloodstream, which burns carbohydrate and fat to supply energy to the body. The human body has more than 600 muscles and 200 bones. Three major systems in the human body relate that are pertinent to aerobic exercise. These include the cardiorespiratory system, the musculoskeletal system, and the nervous system.

- The cardiorespiratory system includes blood, blood vessels, the heart, the lungs, and a series of passageways such as the mouth, throat, trachea, and bronchi. The center of the cardiorespiratory system is the heart.
- The musculoskeletal system includes the bones and the locations and functions of the muscles attached to the skeleton.
- The nervous system is the body's control center and internal communication center. It has three functions:

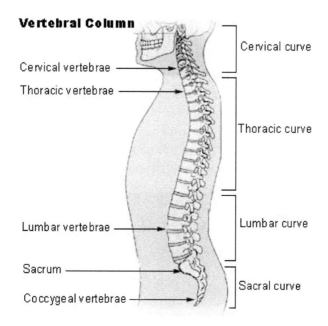

Figure 3.1 Vertebral/spinal column showing the cervical, thoracic, and lumbar regions.

---

    a) It monitors inside and outside body changes;
    b) It formulates body responses by activating muscles or glands;
    c) It analyzes and interprets sensory input to decide what should occur at each and every moment.

The three vertebral regions of the spine—cervical, thoracic, and lumbar (as seen in Figure 3.1)—are very important in African dance, as the head always moves during **90** percent of African cultural dances; African dance is all about body isolations. Specific isolations will be addressed in a later chapter. These isolations, seen in Figure 3.2, take place on three primary planes of action: the sagittal plane, which divides the body into the right and left sides; the frontal, or coronal, plane, which divides the body into the front and back portions; and the transverse plane, which divides the body into the upper and lower portions. All three planes meet at the center of gravity of the body, where almost all the dances start and end.

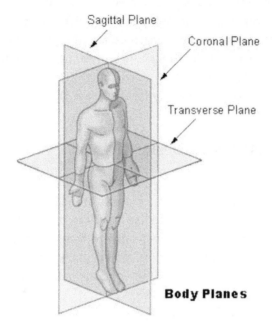

Figure 3.2 Body plane showing the three planes of action: sagittal, frontal/coronal, and transverse.

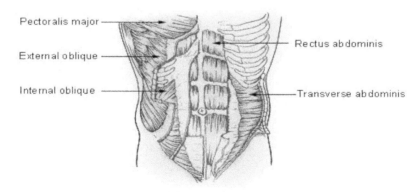

Figure 3.3 A cross-section of the body showing the abdominal muscles.

The stomach, or core, also known as the abdominals, along with the sides or obliques noticeably benefit from African dance because it focuses directly on the abdominal muscles, which are used throughout all the movements of the dances. African dance firms and tones your stomach muscles deeper and more effectively, due to the depth of your pelvic tilt, your boombsey (see Figure 3.3).

DANCE INJURY AND PREVENTION

Safety and injury prevention is an important aspect of African dance. First-timers might feel some muscle pain in their necks, as that is one of the key parts of the body we use in African dance. Also, they might feel some muscle pain in their quads and hamstrings because of the low position of most of the dance moves. Lastly, muscle pain might be felt in the lower back, due to the constant pelvic tilting movements such as moving their boombseys.

To keep the Body from Injury:

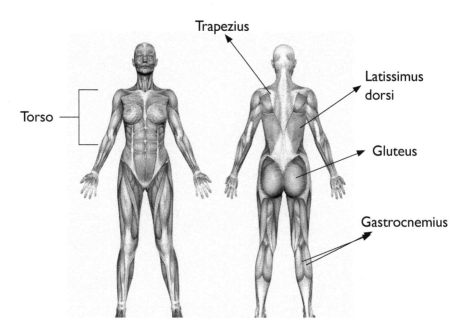

Figure 3.4 Anterior and posterior female muscular system.

Class starts with a thorough warm-up, including stretching, which brings warm blood to the muscles and tendons, making them more pliable and less prone to injury.

Make sure you stretch from head to toe.

- Start with the head, neck, shoulders, arms, and upper body, which houses your trapezius, rhomboids, latissimus dorsi, torso, and oblique muscles
- Finish off with the lower body, which includes the pelvis, gluteus (boombsey), hips, quadriceps or hamstrings, gastrocnemius, and ankles

Emergency Procedures: RICE Treatment Method

When injuries occur, it is important to administer emergency procedures that will facilitate proper recovery. RICE is an acronym for a treatment method recommended for these injuries.

- **R**est is required when injury occurs to any area of the body, thus requiring you to stay in bed. Discontinue stress to the injured area for approximately 24 hours, to allow healing and to prevent reinjury. Following recovery, ease back gently into exercise, and be careful not to attempt too much too soon.
- **I**ce constricts the blood vessels, thus controlling swelling and curbing the pain. Ice also numbs nerve endings, slows blood flow through the broken tissue membranes, and lowers the temperature of the affected area. This method retards inflammation and helps to reduce recovery time. Apply ice as soon as injury occurs. Wrap ice in a towel or plastic bag, or use ready ice packs. Do not apply ice directly to your skin to avoid frostbite. Apply ice every 15 to 20 minutes, changing position every five minutes. Ice should be applied repeatedly for the first 12 hours, to shorten the duration and severity of bleeding and swelling.
- **C**ompression blocks the blood from seeping into the surrounding tissues and ensures that there is no additional swelling. Wrap elastic bandages around the injured area and leave on for about 30 minutes, then remove for about 15 minutes to ensure adequate circulation. Do not wrap too tightly to avoid causing

restricted blood flow or discomfort. Compression should be applied for 48 to 72 hours.

- **E**levation limits swelling by draining excess fluid from the injured area.

Decreasing the swelling can prevent the quantity of injury byproducts that will require removal when healing begins (such as blood clots, etc.). Periodically, position the injured body part above the level of the nearest joint. Elevation can be used in conjunction with ice and compression. Continue elevation, even while sleeping.

Common movement injuries can result from a single impact or from overuse of the muscles, due to cumulative **microtrauma** or **macrotrauma** or both. Microtrauma is pain caused as a result of microtears, and macrotrauma is injury caused from a major source. It is important to know the cause of the injury so that upon returning to activity, the stress that originally caused the injury is not repeated.

Common Injuries That May Occur Due to Improper Execution of Dances:

- Muscle cramp: muscles not stretched or warmed-up
- Hamstring pull: muscles cramping due to tightness
- Shin splints: pain on front or side of legs
- Sore muscles: overuse of muscles
- Side stitch: muscles not stretched or warmed-up
- Iliotibial band Syndrome: incorrect hip stance
- Knee injuries: pain in cartilage of kneecap
- Chondromalacia: grating and pain around kneecap

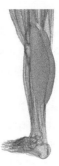

Figure 3.5 Calf muscle

- Meniscus tears: sharp twisting movement of the knee
- Stress fracture :   overuse of bone
- Plantar fascitis: pain in sole of foot
- Tendonitis: pain in calf/leg
- Strain: tear or stretch in muscle/tendon unit
- Sprain: tear in knee or ankle - ligament/joint
- Metatarsalgia: pain in ball of foot
- Bursitis: friction in knees, hip, shoulders, elbows
- Heat injuries: heat cramps, heat exhaustion, heat stroke
- Lower back problems: poor posture, inflexibility of trunk
- Scoliosis: curvature of the spine
- Kyphosis or Sciatica: outward thoracic curve
- Lordosis: exaggerated curve of lower back

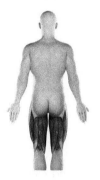

Figure 3.6 Hamstring

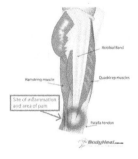

Figure 3.7 Iliotibial band syndrome

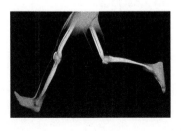

Figure 3.8 Knee injuries

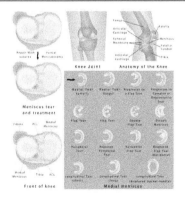

Figure 3.9 Meniscus tears

Heat Injuries

During African dance classes, it is important to take water breaks frequently. If your body is allowed to overheat, heat injuries may occur.

There are three main forms of heat injury:

1. **Heat cramps** are characterized by extremely painful muscular pains and spasms and profuse sweating. Heat cramps do not respond to massage or stretching without immediate treatment.

Treatment

- Move patient to a cooler place
- Dilute the blood by having the patient drink at least four ounces of water every 15 minutes for one hour, then massage the cramps away

2. **Heat exhaustion** is a more serious heat injury characterized by weakness, profuse sweating, pale, clammy skin, and collapse.

Treatment

- Move patient to a cooler place
- Have patient lie down, elevating the feet 8" to 12" higher than the body and loosening clothing
- Cool patient by fanning, splashing with water, and/or applying ice packs
- Obtain medical care as soon as possible

3. **Heat stroke** is the most serious heat injury and can be fatal. The body temperature is extremely high, with no further sweating; the skin is hot and dry; pulse is strong and rapid; pupils are dilated; blood pressure is low. The patient may be unconscious.

Treatment

- Move patient to a cool place
- Remove clothing immediately
- Cool immediately by any means available, e.g., water, ice, fanning
- Continue cooling the body until medical care arrives; waiting may result in brain damage or death

Plantar Fasciitis

Plantar fasciitis is an inflammation of the arch fascia (connective tissue). The fascia acts as a ligament, running from the bottom of the heel, across the foot, and connecting with the toes.

When the arch tries to flatten to accommodate the impact of jumping or stamping the foot, the fascia can become inflamed and even tear. This can also be accompanied by a heel spur, which is a calcium deposit on the bottom of the heel where the ligament attaches to the bone.

People with high arches are more susceptible.

Treatment

- Rest, ice, compression, and elevation (RICE)
- Massage and stretch the arch by rolling it back and forth on a tennis ball; this stimulates blood flow and helps loosen adhesions

Prevention

- Avoid high-impact movements
- Use flexible arch supports or tape the arches
- Wear shoes with both good arch support and flexibility at the balls of the feet
- A sports podiatrist may recommend a cast, special shoe, or device to redistribute force into the arch
- Since the plantar fascia is a continuation of the calf muscle system, arch pain responds to calf and Achilles tendon stretches

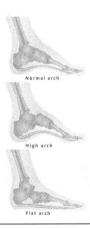

Normal arch

High arch

Flat arch

Figure 3.10 Plantar fascia

Shin Splints

When the feet hit the ground, the sudden impact radiates up the leg bones, with most of the shock being absorbed by the tibialis muscles. Shin splints can involve injury to the muscle, tendon, or bone.

Causes

- Shin splints can result from a muscle imbalance between the tibialis anterior and the gastrocnemius and soleus
- Overuse can cause muscle fibers to swell and even tear
- Inadequate shock absorption can also contribute
- Weak or injured anterior tibialis muscles and tight calf muscles may be responsible

Anterior Shin Splints

Anterior compartment syndrome: The muscles, nerves, and blood vessels of the lower leg are divided into four compartments. During vigorous activity, the anterior compartment can swell, causing the fascia to become tight and create pressure, reducing circulation to the leg.

Surgery is often required to release the fascia. Symptoms include numbness on top of the foot and tenderness over the anterior tibialis for middle shin splint pain, or an achy feeling in the front of the leg for bottom shin splint pain.

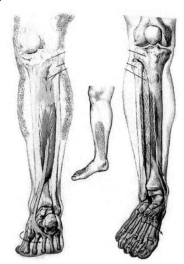

Figure 3.11 Shin splints

Posterior Shin Splints

This involves the posterior tibialis and flexor digitorum longus muscles, the main foot stabilizers. Symptoms include instability, either due to biomechanical imbalance or muscle weakness, and are characterized by pain around the inside of the tibia.

Treatment

- Shin splints should NOT be ignored. Once irritated, the tibial muscles can become rather swollen and press on nerves, causing shooting pain during exercise. RICE should be applied
- In severe cases, complete rest to the injured area is recommended
- Wrap the injured area so the muscle is closer to the bone, or wear supportive hose for additional comfort

Prevention

- Warm up thoroughly, including calf muscle stretches
- Use correct shoes with adequate shock absorption; add insoles if necessary
- Avoid high-impact movements on hard surfaces
- Do not land on the toes; roll the foot all the way through to distribute shock
- Anyone with structural misalignment should consult an orthopedist for further prevention

Side Stitch

Side stitches produce sharp pain on the lower, lateral side of the thoracic wall, the rib cage. The primary cause is spasm, either in the diaphragm or in the muscles between the ribs, produced by improper breathing and lack of oxygen.

Treatment

- Slow down during transitional changes of exercise to bring relief
- Stretch side to relieve discomfort

Prevention

- Warm up thoroughly
- Avoid eating just before exercise

- Avoid gulping water
- Stop during exercise to drink
- Make transitional changes in rate and/or speed gradually

Sore Muscles

Sore muscles result from **microtears** within the muscle itself or in the connective tissue harness that links the tissue to the adjacent bone. Symptoms are swelling, fluid retention, and stiffness in the surrounding tissues and general soreness, also low-level chronic muscle spasms.

Treatment

- Ice
- Rest
- Exercises cause the muscle fibers to increase in size and strength, thus enabling muscles to repair more quickly
- Exercising also stimulates blood flow to the sore muscles, speeding up healing by nourishing the recovering cells and increasing circulation

Prevention

- Always take time to warm up adequately
- Avoid **ballistic stretching**, a quick stretching of a muscle beyond its normal range
- Don't attempt exercising too much or too soon to the point of pain

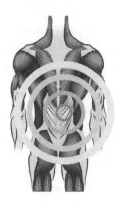

Figure 3.12 Lower back pain

Sprains

Sprains occur when a sudden twist or turn overstretches the ligament, by forcing the joint it supports beyond its normal range of motion. While there is usually no dislocation, sprains result in pain, swelling, and site discoloration. Sprains are also classified according to their severity, with variance in pain, swelling, and disability.

Causes

- Grade 1 sprain: stretching ligament mildly, creating a mild sprain in joint
- Grade 2 sprain: overstretching ligament, creating an intermediate sprain in joint, with mild pain
- Grade 3 sprain: severe stretch of the ligament, creating severe sprain in joint, accompanied by pain, swelling, and disability

Treatment

- Rest
- Ice
- Compression
- Elevation

Prevention

- When executing dance movements, especially on a carpet, use caution.
- See a physician if popping or clicking sounds occur, or if the joint becomes locked in place.

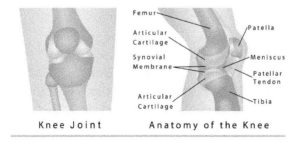

Figure 3.13 Knee joint

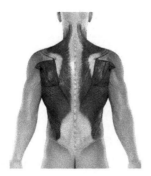

Figure 3.14 Back muscles

Strains

A strain is a muscle microtear that occurs when muscle use exceeds tendon flexibility and strength. Strains are classified according to their severity and most commonly occur in the Achilles tendon, calf, hamstring, and quadriceps areas.

Causes

- Grade I strain: stretching tendon or muscle fibers with a minimum tear
- Grade 2 strain: stretching tendon or muscle fibers, with partial tear accompanied by pain and swelling
- Grade 3 strain: extensive tear of tendon or muscle fibers, with pain, swelling, and indentation at the area of the strain

Treatment

- Rest.
- Ice
- Resume activity slowly and gently, exercising just enough to increase blood flow to the injury site. This can help speed healing by nourishing the recovering cells and encouraging circulation

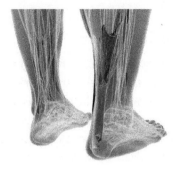

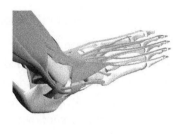

Figure 3.15 Tendinitis   **Figure 3.16** Tendons and ligaments

Prevention

- Do not exercise to the point of pain
- Do not attempt too much too soon
- Do not neglect flexibility training
- Avoid ballistic stretching

In all cases of injury or potential injury, proper medical attention is recommended as an important part of responsible follow-up.

NUTRITION AND HYDRATION

These fabulous physical bodies you each possess run on a certain kind of fuel—food. When you put the proper fuel into your body, it runs efficiently, but when you put in the wrong fuel, it does not run properly. It is that basic and simple!

When you experience physical breakdown, it is merely the body responding to the wrong fuel. Most physical problems we experience, whether it be being over- or underweight, high blood pressure, diabetes, pimples, and the like is merely the body reacting to the wrong fuel.

For your body to be in harmony when performing African dances, it is essential to feed and hydrate it correctly.

Nutritional Needs for Dance

The best nutrition for such vibrant dancing is to eat more roughage, fruits, and vegetables to build your strength to enable you to perform at your utmost. Eat moderately of predominantly living foods and plant-based foods. Avoid junk foods and snack on healthy foods such as unsalted cashews, sunflower seeds, carrots, celery, broccoli, and sweet peppers. Do not eat after 9 P.M. Your metabolism slows down tremendously by the end of your day, thus making it hard to digest the food at late hours before you go to bed. Drink clean purified water every day, and if you have not already done so, switch to fruit and vegetable drinks from soft drinks, to help build your cells. Eat more fresh fruits and vegetables. Each fruit and vegetable supplies vitamins which your body needs. Africans cook from scratch and they cook fresh each day, as they feed large families and need to have enough to go around.

Get as much fresh air as possible—it is good for your lungs. If weather permits, enjoy the sunlight as well. Do not wear sunglasses all the time. Your eyes need the full spectrum of the sun to be healthy.

Healthy Juicing Combinations

Juicing is another form of providing ample nutrients to your body. The following juicing combinations are listed with their potential benefits.

- **Carrot + Ginger + Apple**—Boost and cleanse your system
- **Apple + Cucumber + Celery**—Prevent cancer, reduce cholesterol, and eliminate stomach upset and headache
- **Tomato + Carrot + Apple**—Improve skin complexion and eliminate bad breath
- **Bitter gourd + Apple + Nut Milk**—Avoid bad breath and reduce internal body heat
- **Orange + Ginger + Cucumber**—Improve skin texture and moisture and reduce body heat
- **Pineapple + Apple + Watermelon**—Dispel excess salts; nourish the bladder and kidneys
- **Apple + Cucumber + Kiwi**—To improve skin complexion

- **Pear + Banana**—Regulate sugar content
- **Carrot + Apple + Pear + Mango**—Clear body heat, counteract toxicity, decrease blood pressure, and fight oxidization
- **Honeydew + Grape + Watermelon + Nut Milk**—Rich in vitamin C + Vitamin B2, which increase cell activity and strengthen body immunity
- **Papaya + Pineapple + Nut Milk**—Rich in vitamins C, E, and iron. Improve skin complexion and metabolism
- **Banana + Pineapple + Nut Milk**—Rich in vitamin with nutrients; prevent constipation

As an African dance student, you will need to prepare your body to be able to endure the rigor, as well as the resulting benefits. The nutritional information given and the combination of juicing fruits and vegetables will help you fortify your body for a healthy lifestyle. Dr. Paul Malkmus of Hallelujah Acres provides nutritional facts throughout his website to help you better understand how your body functions (http://www.hacres.com/).

Hydration

An exercising body produces heat, which is normally dissipated by the sweating process. During hot weather, your body can lose too much water from sweating. This problem is amplified in high humidity, when the air is already saturated with water vapor and is unable to absorb enough sweat to adequately cool the body. This causes the heart to pump harder in an attempt to carry more blood to the skin for cooling. More sweat is produced, but is ineffective in cooling the body. In the process, so much water is lost that the blood becomes thickened, further straining the heart, blocking oxygen delivery to the internal tissues, and elevating core temperature. The effect on the tissues and organs is as hot as an oven. It is essential to take water breaks when dancing.

Even during cold climates, dancing in a hot studio will deem it necessary to stay hydrated.

SHORT-TERM AND LONG-TERM BENEFITS OF AFRICAN DANCE

You will begin to reap some short-term physical benefits that will be apparent in a short period of time. In addition, you will gain some significant long-term benefits as you continue your dance classes.

The Short-Term Physical Benefits of African Dance Include Improvements to the Following Areas:

- Cardiovascular endurance and respiratory systems
- Efficiency of body performance
- Muscle flexibility and cardiac efficiency
- Increase in stroke volume—blood that is pumped with each heartbeat
- Lowered heart rate
- Muscular endurance and strength
- Breathing capacity
- Increased capacity of respiratory ventilation
- Capacity for dissipating metabolically produced heat

The Long-Term Physical Benefits of African Dance Include:

- Increase in lean body mass and muscle mass
- Decrease in body fat
- Positive, visible changes in body composition

As you continue in this journey of learning to execute African dances, several improvements to your respiratory and cardiovascular systems will be apparent—improvements such as lowered heart rate, better breathing capacity, and muscular strength. Ultimately, with continued dancing, long-term benefits occur that are exhibited in the visible changes you will notice in your body composition.

Summary

Several factors must be considered when undertaking African dance. The studio has to be conducive to dancing barefoot, and your attire should not be restrictive. It is important that you answer certain health questions to ensure that you are healthy enough to start dancing. You have to be cognizant of your body's anatomy and the potential for injury should you not follow instruction. Finally, it is beneficial for your body to be properly hydrated before, during, and after dancing. If you are not currently eating properly, change your diet to include living foods such as fruits and vegetable. Being aware of what is safe and healthy will contribute to a great dancing experience.

Glossary

Aerobic	An exercise the improves the body's utilization of oxygen
Anaerobic	An exercise that does not improve the body's utilization of oxygen
Ballistic stretching	A quick stretching of a muscle beyond its normal range
Kinesiology	The study of human movement
Macrotrauma	An injury from a major source
Microtear	The destruction of micro-filaments in a muscle cell
Microtrauma	The pain caused as a result of microtears

References

Aerobics and Fitness Association of America. (2010). *Fitness & theory practice manual.* Sherman Oaks, CA: AFAA.

Alcamo, E. I. (2004). *Anatomy and physiology the easy way.* Hauppauge, NY: Barron's Educational Series, Inc.

American Council on Exercise. (2008). *Advanced health & fitness specialist manual: The ultimate resource for advanced fitness professionals.* San Diego: ACE.

National Dance Exercise Instructors Training Association. (1990/1999). *Aerobics & fitness instructor's training manual: Fitness manual update.* Minneapolis, MN: NDEITA.

Nuamah, K., (2005). *Kukuwa® dance workout: KDW® instructor training manual* (pp. 16–30). Unpublished Manual.

Thibodeau, G. A., and Patton, K. T. (2011). *Structure & function of the body* (14th ed.), Mosby-Year Books.

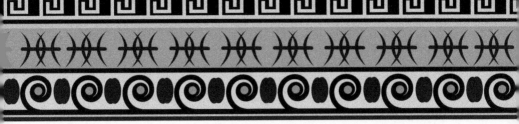

Chapter 4

LEARNING AND PERFORMING THE BASICS OF AFRICAN DANCE

B efore you delve into African dance, it is important to understand how these dances came into being. The stories behind the songs, the tempo of various dances that further define the occasion, and careful movement of several components of the body are all interwoven to form the fabric of the African dance experience.

AFRICAN DANCE AND MUSIC

The underlying premise of African dances is a story that has to be told. These stories stem from various occasions in life. African dance, in concert with the music, presents a pictorial movement of various beliefs, ceremonies, and life events of those particular cultures.

Some of the various influences that form and inform African dances are:

- Conscience collective
- Communal philosophies
- Nature
- History of communities
- Daily experiences*

Dances

Each region of Africa (North, South, East, West, and central) has its own ethnic tribes, and each tribe has its very own authentic dance performances that stand for different occasions and events. There are African dances in Table 4.1 from different countries of the continent and their status:

Table 4.1 Selected African Dances from All Over the Continent

DANCE	EVENT	TRIBE	COUNTRY
Adumu	Coming of Age	Maasai	Kenya
Adzogbu	Ritual War	Ewe	Benin and Ghana
Agahu	Socializing	Egun	Nigeria
Agbekor	War & Funeral	Ewe, Foh	Ghana
Assiko	Relationships	Doula	Cameroon
Atsia	Morality	Ewe	Ghana
Bawa	Harvest	Dagarthi	Northern Ghana
Dipo	Initiation	Krobo	Ghana
Eskesta	Ritual	Amharic	Ethiopia
Eunot	Rite of Passage	Maasai	Kenya
FumeFume	Socializing	Ga	Ghana
Gadzo	Spiritual	Ewe	Ghana
Guerda	Spiritual	Tuareg Berber	Morocco
Indlamu	War/Wedding	Zulu	South Africa
Kpanlogo	Recreation	Ga	Ghana
Mbende	Initiation	Jerusamera	Zimbabwe
Mirobayasa	Cleaning	Malinke	Guinea
Mouwa	Farming	Bambara, Senufo, Minianka	Mali
Muchongoyo	Spiritual	Ndebele	Zimbabwe
Nmane	Wedding	Akan	Ghana
Runyege	Courtship	Batooro	Uganda
Safiatu	Spiritual	Bamiléké	Cameroon
Umteyo	Welcome	Xhosa	South Africa
Sorsorone	Harvest	Baga	Guinea

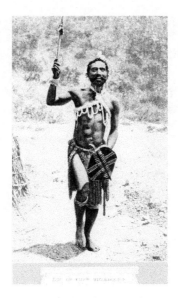

Figure 4.1 Dancer from the Zulu tribe of South Africa.

Beliefs and Worship Dance

Three categories incorporate the events at which African dances are performed: beliefs, ceremonies, and life events. In African cultures, there is always a belief in a higher being. Based on that belief, certain dances are geared toward requests for certain things in life. Some of the requests may be for a bountiful fishing season, a blessing on a marriage, or seeking direction in life. Beliefs and worship can get very deep for the tribes of Africa, and such dances are performed in reverence to both ancestors and other tribes for a pardon of something done wrong or for a request of a favor needed.

Ajayi wrote of the dynamic between African dance and religion: "Dance is undoubtedly a vital means of communicating with the sacred in African religious practices; it is an expressive form fully integrated within the worship system."

Welsh stated this example of a beliefs and worship dance: "The Banda is a Cewa tribal dance from Malawi that is performed in a ceremony to worship Gede, the god of cemeteries and reproduction. The dance symbolizes death and life, as well as the celebration of the future and the past in the present moment."

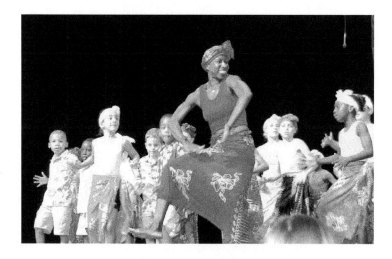

Figure 4.2 Adzohu-Dahomeyan Dance; a stage presentation of West African sacred dance.

Begho wrote about how dancing has been incorporated into worship services: "The most significant innovation in the area of religious dancing that contemporary Africa has witnessed exists in the free African churches known under the generic name, Aladura, in Nigeria. Prior to the appearance of the Aladura churches on the scene of religious worship in Africa and, in fact, a long time after the new churches had gained ground, the orthodox Christian churches of European origin, as well as the Muslim movements of Arabic origin, did not accept dance as an integral part of their religious worship."

According to Sobania, "the adaptation of traditional music and drumming by Roman Catholic churches has helped preserve important musical traditions in many regions" of Kenya.

Essien and Falola stated, "Religious music varies regionally. In the north, most religious ceremonies are accompanied by music. Northern Sudanese music has its roots in haqibah, a type of religious music that emerged in the 1920s. Haqibah is directly linked with madeeh, a form of a cappella music. Haqibah has ties to both European and Egyptian music. Music in the north is also shaped by Arab instruments such as the oud, which provides a distinct melody as musicians play them."

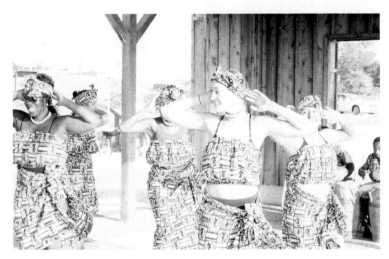

Figure 4.3 Performance of Ekpui ceremony from Ghana.

Welsh wrote specifically about Muslim dancing in Africa: "Whirling Dervishes, known as the Mevlevi Order of Sufi Muslims, practice a devotional dance called the Ritual of Sema in Libya, Sudan, Egypt, Tunis, and Morocco. The ceremony, which can last for hours, represents a spiritual journey; the dancers turn toward God in hope of establishing a greater understanding and union with God."

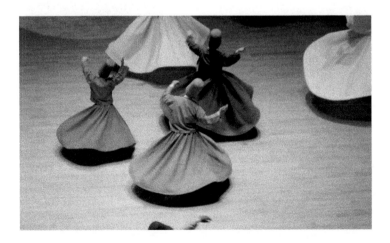

Figure 4.4 Whirling Dervish dancers.

Ceremonial Dances

Ceremonial dances are important in African dances. There are ceremonial dances that depict fighting, weddings, festivals, royalty, and tribal communication. Some of these dances are call-and-response dances, in which one dance is the completion of the other. The two parts of the dance form a complete thought.

Births and initiations are taken very seriously by the African people, and each tribe performs its extensive rituals accordingly. The significance of initiation is the determination of how a child will fare in life; thus the seriousness of it.

Begho wrote of ceremonial dances: "Perhaps the single largest category of traditional African dances is the group termed ceremonial. Two main subdivisions—sectarian and communal—are discernible, and under them come various subcategories. The distinction between the two subdivisions is founded on the assumption that the former deals with those dances which are expressive of the ethos and pathos of an allied group within a community at some particular eventful moment or occasion in the group's collective life. The latter is all-embracing, dealing with those dances which are expressive of the ethos and pathos of the community as a whole as some particular eventful moment in the collective life of the entire community."

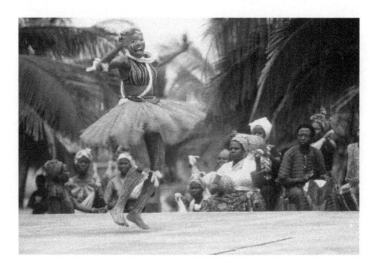

Figure 4.5 Woman performing a ceremonial dance in West Africa.

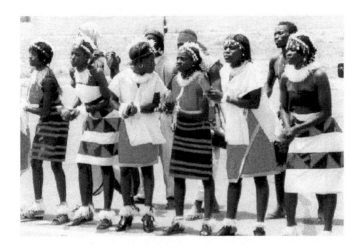

Figure 4.6 People performing a traditional dance in Banjul, The Gambia.

Rites-of-Passage Dances

As with most events in African culture, life events are also celebrated with various significant dances. A rite of passage celebrates a realization of freedom, if you will. This is a dance performed by boys and girls to mark their entry into woman- or manhood. In Ghana, initiation into adult life begins at the age of nine for females and 13 for males.

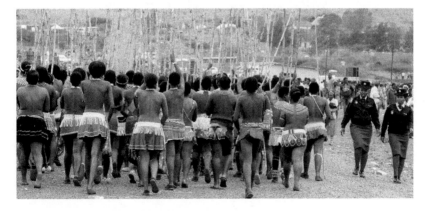

Figure 4.7 Zulu Reed Dance Festival in South Africa

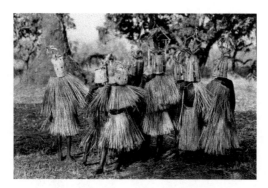

Figure 4.8 Yao boys participating in initiation rites.

The initiates are schooled in the secrets and complexities of life by the older women and men in the community.

According to Welsh, rites-of-passage "dances range from detailed footwork all the way to a swinging of the hips. The aesthetic qualities of the dances vary greatly by ethnic group. These dances often are more than just figurative representations and, for many ethnic groups, suggest an actual change in status from childhood to manhood or womanhood. [They] are almost always gender-specific, with boys dancing with boys and girls dancing with girls."

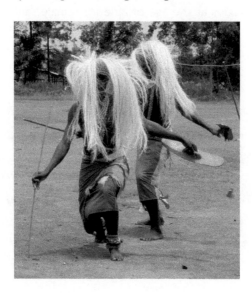

Figure 4.9 Orphaned young men learn a traditional dance near Kigali, Rwanda.

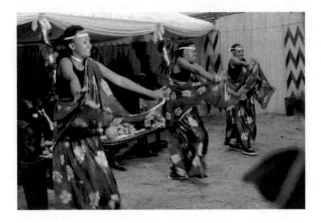

Figure 4.10 Women in Rwanda perform a harvest dance.

Other African Dances

Other African dances include:

- Royal dances
- Children's dances
- War dances
- Fertility dances

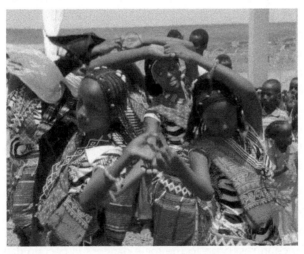

Figure 4.11 Young women perform a traditional African wedding dance in Kontali, Djibouti.

- Harvest dances
- Courtship/moonlight dances
- Funeral dances
- Wedding dances

Dancers

An Akan proverb states that *asare boni nkom asaase*. Translated to English, it means: a bad dance does not kill the earth. The proverb invites all who desire to dance, regardless of their expertise. With that attitude and expression toward dance, male, female, and children alike partake in dancing. Dancing is prevalent in all aspects of African life. The young African child learns to incorporate dancing—ceremonial or recreational—into their lives. As soon as a child is able to walk, she is exposed to dancing and is allowed to partake in all forms of it. Unlike Western cultures, where parties can be specifically for adults, an African child attends most functions with his parents.

Children may be seen in ceremonial dances as early as three years of age in full regalia. Depending on the dance, a headdress may be worn, although this is not always the case. Some dances use tailored outfits, while others use pieces of cloth. Regardless of the form of costume, the male version differs from the female.

Welsh wrote about how societal roles have been utilized: "For the most part, in traditional settings, military, war, and martial arts dances are performed by men, but there are exceptions in some ethnic groups where women participate in or have their own war dances. [In Zimbabwe,] the Zezuru created distractions out of their own resources, namely, women and music. In this way, the Mbende was born. [Zezuru warriors] lined up a group of old men with [drums and other instruments]. When the men began playing the musical instruments, the women would run out onto the field and start dancing. Those too old or too young to fight were sometimes used in Mbende, since they would be perfect decoys."

Female Dancers

Female dancers have specific roles in African dance. For instance, the females dance in response to the male dancers in certain dances, and in others, the females continue the dance that the males have started,

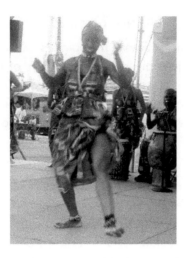

Figure 4.12 Female Adowa dancer from Ghana.

thus creating a complete dance. There is certainly always a female part of the dance and a male part of the dance. At times, some of the dances require both genders to perform the same movement within the actual dance, then back to their own parts of the dance.

Regarding gender roles, Welsh wrote, "Women use dance to convey modesty, grace, and demureness—often to express gender identity."

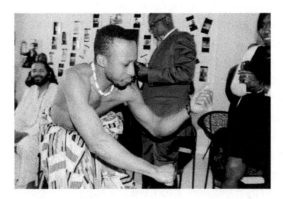

Figure 4.13 Male Adowa dancer from Ghana.

Male Dancers

Male dancers are almost always the starters of the dance, thus inviting the females to join the dance. Their part of the dance is very vibrant and carries a lot of strength movements that can usually only be performed by the males. In African society, the male is the head of the family, and this is also depicted in the dances performed by males.

Dance Costumes

African dances do not have a standard costume because different dances require different outfits, even within the same tribe. The outfits contribute to the essence of the stories being told. Different costumes also speak to the various regions from which these dances have emerged. Even though students in African dance classes will not be dressed in the traditional costumes of the dances they will be learning, it is important to be aware of those costumes.

Male dancers tend to be outfitted in more masculine regalia. The cloth for the male for the Adowa dance is tied around the waist and folded over to secure it. The chest is bare, except for the jewelry around the neck. The arms and wrists are adorned with jewelry for males, and the dancer wears a headpiece as well. Jewelry for a male is bigger and bolder than jewelry for females and is traditionally 24-karat gold. A variation of the costume for elderly and royal males is to have them wrapped loosely around and tossed over the left shoulder. The cloth for a male is larger than that for a female, measuring about five yards.

The female regalia are usually demure as compared to the male. If pieces of cloth are used, as in the case of the Adowa dance of Ghana, the female ties the first cloth on the bottom to form a skirt. The second piece of cloth is wrapped around the torso and folded over, all around the chest to secure it. There is also a third, smaller piece of material that is tied around the waist. Around the neck, arms, wrists, and ankles of the female dancer is jewelry, which traditionally is 24-karat gold. With Ghana being a gold mining country, no expense is spared when it comes to this regal dance. A variation of this outfit for elderly and royal women is to have the top piece loosely wrapped around the torso and tossed over the left shoulder. The head of the dancer also has a piece that looks like a headband.

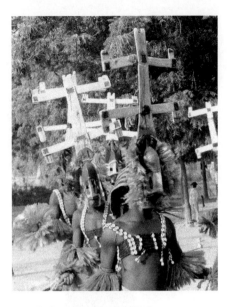

Figure 4.14 Dogon mask dance in Sangha, Mali.

Finally, it is essential to mention that the children are dressed as mini-adult males and females.

Regarding the importance of costumes, Warren wrote, "In many dances, the movements are determined by the costumes. The whirling turns of the Taki dance make wide billowing shapes of the dancers full-flowing smocks."

Welsh wrote about costumes and masks: "The dance of the Bou Saada is from Tunisia and is danced by women. They sing in couplets alternately in Sudanese dialect and wear costumes that have multicolored paper crowns and skirts made up of reeds, feathers, and shells.

Mask dances are dances that utilize a mask and/or a full-body covering that conceals and hides the identity of the dancers so that the focus is on the figure. The Midimu (mask dancers), who are from the Makonde tribe of southern Tanzania and Mozambique, dance during the rites of boys and girls coming out of the respective initiation camps. The Mozambique Makonde Midimu mask is much like a helmet, covering the entire head and won at an angle, slanting backwards to allow air circulation through the neck end of the mask the mouth, eyes, and of course, the nostrils."

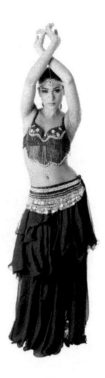

Figure 4.15 Arabic belly dancer.

Dance Events

Dancing occurs during celebrations such as birthdays, weddings, accomplishments, and graduations or for entertainment such as cultural dance troupe performances, or for festivals such as the Bakatue, the celebration for the opening of the fishing season. Regarding celebrations in Kenya, Sobania wrote that, "weddings almost always include song and dance, as do festivities that include processions." Welsh noted that, "The Baladi [Egyptian belly dancing] is performed at weddings, birthdays, parties, and public festivals such as the Mawalid or Saints' Days."

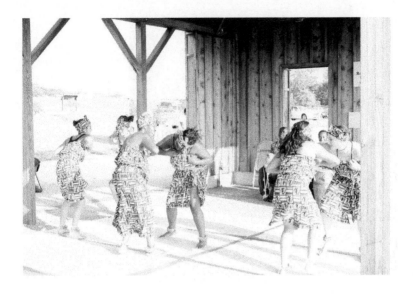

Figure 4.16 Performance of Kpanlogo dance from Ghana.

Celebrations

When celebrating birthdays, accomplishments, weddings, and the like, the songs are contemporary. The dances performed at these occasions are personalized with undertones of tradition. It is not unusual for people to rush the floor at the start of the song *Kpanlogo Yε De*, which translated means Kpanlogo is enjoyable. They may not perform the traditional kpanlogo dance throughout the song, but would place their own spin on the execution of it. If someone appears to be performing exceptionally, others will surround and fan their handkerchiefs while verbally encouraging the dancer. It is not unusual at these functions to see two females dancing together or a group of women. The sense of community is exhibited by this behavior with no underlying connotation. Men, women, and children dance together, and no one needs an invitation to be on the dance floor.

As Begho put it, "Little wonder, then that there usually are as many different dances as there are individuals on the dance floor. To be sure it is the improvisational genius of some fans and, sometimes,

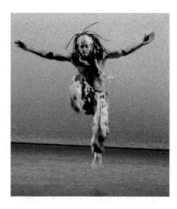

Figure 4.17 Nimba, a traditional dance of the Malinke from Guinea and Mali.

the popular musicians themselves to credit for a good number of vogue dances."

Entertainment

When it comes to dances for entertainment of the public, these dances are strictly traditional and are accompanied by drums. The dances that are performed at cultural centers or by dance troupes are very traditional and precise. Stories are conveyed that have been passed on from generation to generation. In Ghana, West Africa, for instance, performances such as the Kpanlogo, Abagja, and Adowa, to name a few, are performed in unison in precise movements. The dancers listen to the changes and tempo of the drumming to cue movement changes. The male and female portions are executed flawlessly. This form of dancing is what you will strive to achieve as a student of African dance.

Welsh wrote that, "Dances are performed in both traditional and contemporary settings, such as a nightclub. [The Baladi is] performed in clubs, hotels, and theaters and is usually part of a larger program of entertainment." Begho mused, "The increasing detachment of the present generation from the hitherto binding traditional social customs has not left dance unaffected. It has led to the adaptation of a very good number of traditional dances that once served more serious uses for entertainment purposes with or without remunerative motive."

Festivals

Festivals are infused in all aspects of African culture. Festivals are specific to a tribe and are presented with much fanfare. Festivals exist for the beginning of the fishing season, Christmas, Easter, and more. One such festival is the Bakatue. The festival is celebrated in the central region of Ghana to officially open the fishing season and literally means "the opening of the lagoon." The festival starts with a gathering of chiefs, queen mothers, and their entourage. There is drumming and dancing alongside the 24-karat-gold–clad chiefs, who are carried to the festival. Praises are given while the entourage dances until all chiefs are seated. Additionally, following the pouring of libation to ancestors, there are several dances that are performed by groups, as well as canoe races. This festival occurs the first Tuesday in July. According to Sobania, "The annual Kenya Music Festival competition takes place each August between the country's secondary schools."

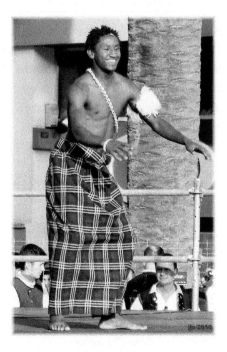

Figure 4.18 Dancer performing at a folklore festival in Kenya.

Some Other Dance Festivals in Africa

Ghanaian Dance Festivals

http://www2.gsu.edu/~finjws/emmat4.htm

South African Dance Festivals

http://www.southafrica.info/travel/cultural/festivals.htm#.UwUXZG3n_IU

Nigerian Dance Festivals

http://www.onlinenigeria.com/festivals/

Asa Bakoo

http://www.sponsume.com/project/asa-baako-music-and-dance-festival-ghana

Dance Umbrella

http://danceumbrella.co.za/home/dance-umbrella-background.html

Zindala Zombili African Music & Dance Festival

https://www.facebook.com/zindalafestival?filter=2

African Dance, Drums, and Drumming

In most African dances, the relationship between the drummer and the dancer is pivotal. The drums call to the dancer, and she, in turn, responds with the appropriate steps. Throughout the dance, the dancer is in harmony with the beats from the drum. Dancing can extend the performance if the drummer senses exuberance and continues to respond with louder melodic strikes. There is no counting in African dancing, so listening to the rhythms of the drums is very important in order to keep to the downbeat. It can be easy, but it can also be challenging. A change in dance movement

Table 4.2 Selected African Music and Dances and Their Countries of Origin

African Music/Dance	Country of Origin
Hi-Life	Ghana
Soukous	Democratic Republic of the Congo
Juju and Fuji	Nigeria
Makossa	Cameroon
Zglibithy	Côte d'Ivoire
Mbalax	Senegal
Taarab	East Africa
Zulu	South Africa

is signified by a change in the tempo of the drums, a change in the pattern of the beat, or a change in the loudness of the drums. After several lessons, these are cues that a student of African dance will learn to recognize and be able to instinctively change dance movements. It is important, therefore, that you pay attention to instruction in order to learn the movements and techniques of African dance. You have to pay close attention to the teacher to be able to duplicate the movements and to pick up on guidance for cues. Students will need to listen closely to the drummer in conjunction with observing the instructor, as the two work in synergy.

African Dance

Today's music and dancing, however, is a mixture of the traditional and modern African sounds. Table 4.2 shows a list of these traditionally influenced modern dances and their countries of origin. You will be exposed to these songs and dances as a student of African dance, even though dance in class is performed mainly with drums.

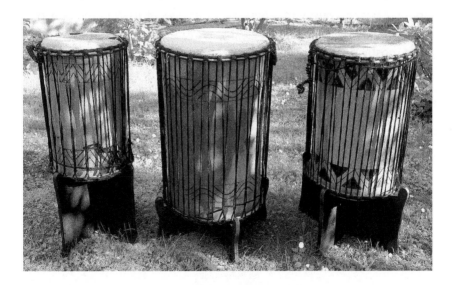

Figure 4.19 D'jun D'jun drum.

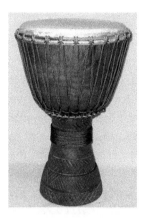

Figure 4.20 D'jimbe drum.

African Drums

Drums are an essential part of many African dances. The sounds of each drum are unique to that particular style. The names of some drums were derived from the sound produced when struck. In addition to providing the beats to dances, drums are used for communication. When someone of importance such as royalty dies, drums are used in some tribes to convey the message. Drums were used in the past to warn of impending danger. Today, those drum patterns still exist, but have mostly been incorporated into dance. There is still, however, the announcement of the death of royalty by drumbeats.

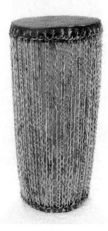

Figure 4.21 Dondo drum.

Below are examples of drums that are indigenous to some regions in Africa:

D'JUN D'JUN—A large double-headed drum, used to keep the traditional orchestra's tempo. The tempo dictates the speed of the dance in accordance with the orchestra, either fast or slow. It is played with a thick stick about two inches in diameter, but can also be played along with the hand.

D'JIMBE—The d'jimbe is a champagne glass–shaped drum, carved with a single piece of wood and played with the hands. The d'jimbe is the lead solo instrument and melody drum in the orchestra.

DONDO or TAMMA (Small Talking Drum)—This is an hourglass-shaped drum with animal skin on both ends, connected by strings that are flexible to tighten or loosen the heads on the drum to create different sounds. The Dondo or Tamma is a drum used to relay messages to the village people (as in public announcements). African languages are tone derived; meanings are given to words with different sounds. The drum is placed under the arm, and the drummer speaks by squeezing the strings with his arm as he plays, changing the tones that create words and phrases.

BREKETE (Large Talking Drum)—This instrument is played two or more at a time. It is a bigger-type drum, the shape of a larger conga,

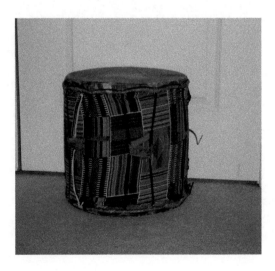

Figure 4.22 Brekete drum.

and has hand carvings on the side and animal skin on the top of it. It is a loud drum, and its sound travels quite a distance when played. It is also used to relay messages to the village people.

Almost every region of Africa has its own particular drums that might not be common to the rest of the continent. The drums are usually made by hand, and some of the materials used to build them are wood and animal skin. Welsh mentioned that in Malawi, "a msondo drum is used—one end only is covered with goatskin—which is struck by the player's hands."

Nketia noted that, "The distribution of drums of particular design and construction tends to be restricted to limited geographical areas. The Ugandan drum, for example is peculiar to eastern Africa. Outside of Uganda, versions of it are found in Ethiopia, as well as in Kenya and Burundi. Similarly, other varieties of small hand drums are found in different parts of eastern Africa."

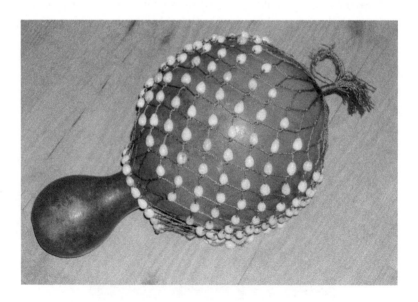

Figure 4.23 Achin.

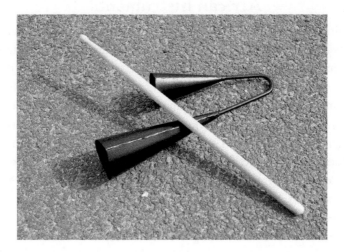

Figure 4.24 Dahur.

Welsh explained that in North Africa, "Vumi, a large bass drum and capuo drums, which are cylindrical in shape and covered with goatskin on both ends, are played during the performance along with brass vitasa cymbals, and a zumari clarinet."

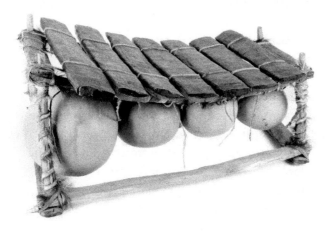

Figure 4.25 Balaphone.

African Instruments

In addition to drums, other instruments are used to augment the melody of the beats for the dancer. These instruments provide unique tones and are great for highlighting certain parts of the stories during dancing. During the Adowa dance, for instance, the sound of the bell will cause the female dancers to dance on their tiptoes and raise their hands a little higher. Most of the instruments are made of household material that allows them to produce certain peculiar sounds that one does not hear outside of the continent. The materials stem from the bark of a tree, to the stems of a plant, to the actual fruit dried up, to seeds, beads, pebbles, sticks, and stones.

ACHIN or SHEKERE (Maracas)—A rattle instrument made from a gourd, which in Africa grows on trees, with beads strung on the outside that rattles when shaken. A melodic instrument which provides a different type of tempo to the orchestra and to the dancers.

DAHUR (Cowbell)—This is a metal instrument in the shape of a bell. Some are two- or three-headed and others have only one. Each head makes a different sound, which usually dictates the step of the dancers in rhythm.

BALAPHONE (Xylophone)—An instrument made of wood, having several keys of different pitch. The larger wood is a lower tone, and the smaller wood is a higher tone.

Other Instruments Used in Africa (Definitions from Wikipedia):

An **idiophone** is any musical instrument which creates sound primarily by way of the instrument's vibrating, without the use of strings or membranes.

A **chordophone** is any musical instrument that makes sound by way of a vibrating string or strings stretched between two points.

A **membranophone** is any musical instrument which produces sound primarily by way of a vibrating stretched membrane.

An **aerophone** is any musical instrument that produces sound primarily by causing a body of air to vibrate, without the use of strings or membranes, and without the vibration of the instrument itself adding considerably to the sound.

AFRICAN DANCE BODY MOVEMENTS

Unlike Western dances, African dances are not universal. Body movements are specific to each dance. You will experience the movement of at least five individual components of your body. For each dance, you will learn the movements of the legs and feet, the arms, the head and neck, and the torso and pelvis. No dance is taught in this particular sequence, as the dances are always taught via breakdown sequence with whichever part of the body that is easiest to move first. As mentioned before, every dance is different. Sometimes the top is taught before the bottom, and vice versa. There is no standard across African dances. The movements of the dances are sometimes natural imitations of animals, birds, reptiles, and wildlife, and also of daily work activities of the people, which signify gracefulness, beauty, strength, bravery, and intelligence. The rhythms of the drums are also obtained from watching and studying the wonders of nature and the essence of life. The dances and the drumming are passed down from generation to generation to the children as early as the age of two or three, when the child can comprehend.

Legs and Feet

There are several movements of the legs and feet of which the student of African dance should be aware. Since each dance has its own unique movements, this serves as an overall description of some of the basic movements you can expect to perform. Individual movements are part of a whole dance that are named differently, depending on the region. It would be difficult to give an ethnic name for a particular movement. One movement is to start on the heel and then flip to the toes. This movement is simply called heel-toe. This is repeated as the dance requires. Another movement is moving the feet one, two, then double move on the feet again. This is simply called single-single-double-double. Another movement would be to bend the leg at the knee while hopping on the other foot. If you are flexible, you will be able to bend your leg until your heel touches your bottom. This movement is simply called heel to boombsey.

Another movement will be to place one foot in front of the other while bending at the waist and slowly walking forward—simply called

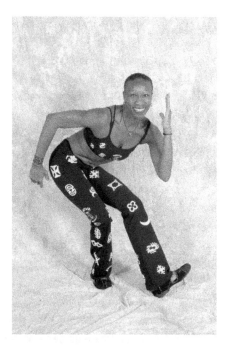

Figure 4.26 Leg and heel movement.

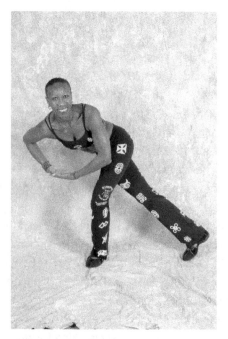

Figure 4.27 Leg and foot movements.

baby steps. Still another motion is to step back with your right leg, then immediately step forward on the same foot, then simultaneously step on the left leg, then immediately step forward on the same foot. This is simply called "one-two-three-step, one-two-three-step." A different sequence is to begin moving the right foot forward, then follow it with the left foot right next to it; then you begin to turn all the way around to the left by pivoting the feet all the way. Do the same with the opposite direction left, and pivot the feet all the way until back to front of the room. This is simply called *kwa wo ho*. Chapter 6 will showcase individual dances and how these types of movements fit into the choreography.

Arms

The arms are a huge part of the storytelling of these dances and help differentiate one movement from another. The hands may be positioned above the head, either clasped or unclasped. They may be positioned to the side, above the knees, by the ankles, around the waist, behind the head, on the shoulders, in front of the chest, bent at the elbow while being flapped, and bent at the elbow and pressed toward each other. Arm movements are too numerous to generalize and will be covered with the specific dance in Chapter 6.

Head and Neck

You will realize how important the head and neck are to African dance. It is an expressive dance, but unlike Western dances that keep the head still, a lot of African dances—to which you will be exposed—require that the head be moved forward and backward. This is done simultaneously with other parts of the body. The head always follows the direction of the arms in the African dance. If the dance movement has the arms going toward the right, then the head goes in the same direction. Some students find they must ease into this movement because they are slightly dizzy. By the end of the class, every student is able to execute this move with confidence.

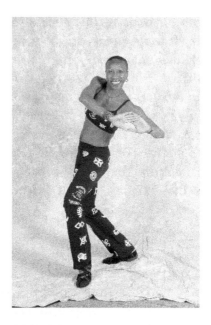

Figure 4.28 Head movement.

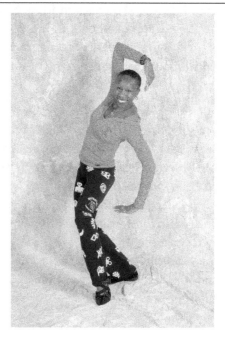

Figure 4.29 Arm movement.

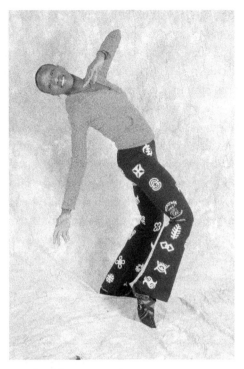

Figure 4.30 Torso and pelvis movement.

Torso and Pelvis

This combination of body parts contributes to the aesthetics of African dance. The torso and pelvis are moved forward and back, side to side, and even in a circular motion. You will be taught dances where, within a second, the torso and pelvis will have been moved three times in rapid succession. This seems nearly impossible to the new student, but with observation of the instructor and understanding of the drumming, you will be able to perform this better than when first instructed. You should realize that not everyone will master these movements.

Overall, African dance is compiled of isolations of the body from the head all the way down to the feet. As mentioned earlier, the body moves anywhere from two to five components at a time.

While learning the basic techniques of African dance, you will be exposed to the various stories that are the premise of these dances. Although dancing in class will be accompanied by drums, it is important to know the various types of music that originated from across the continent and how modern variations have influenced these dances. African dancing occurs at events for celebrations, entertainment, and festivals. The dances for celebrations are modernized, and those performed at festivals and for entertainment are traditional in execution. The progression of dance that you will encounter as an African dance student will start with techniques for the legs and feet, the arms, head and neck, and then torso and pelvis. Several drums are used to accompany performances, and some of these names are derived by the sounds created. Finally, it is important to differentiate the clothing and roles of male and female dancers. Children are dressed as mini-adults and can participate in dance troops as early as age two or three.

GLOSSARY

Abagja	A festive dance performed by the Ewe tribe of Ghana, West Africa
Achin (Shekere)	A rattle instrument made from a gourd, which in Africa grows on trees, with beads strung on the outside that rattle when shaken
Adowa	A regal dance performed by the Akan people in Ghana, West Africa
Akan	The tribe that occupies the southern part of Ghana and speaks variations of the Akan language
Balaphone	An instrument made of wood, having several keys of different pitch
Brekete	A large drum, shaped as a Conga with hand carvings on the side and animal skin on the top
Dahur	A metal instrument in the shape of a bell
D'jimbe	A champagne glass–shaped drum, carved with a single piece of wood and played with the hands
D'jun D'jun	A large double-headed drum, used to keep the traditional orchestra's tempo

Dondo (Tamma) An hourglass-shaped drum with animal skin on both ends, connected by strings that are flexible to tighten or loosen the heads on the drum, thereby creating different sounds

Kpanlogo A dance performed by the Ga tribe of Ghana, West Africa

Safiatu A belief and worship dance from Cameroon

REFERENCES

Begho, F. (1996). *Traditional dance in African dance*, from *African dance: An artistic, historical, and philosophical inquiry* (K. Welsh Asante, Ed.). Trenton, NJ: Africa World Press, Inc.

Essien, K., and Falola, T. (2009). *Culture and customs of Sudan.* Westport, CT: Greenwood Press.

Nketia, J. H. K. (1974). *The music of Africa.* New York: W. W. Norton & Company, Inc.

Sobania, N. (2003). *Culture and customs of Kenya.* Westport, CT: Greenwood Press.

Warren, L. (1972). *The dance of Africa.* Englewood Cliffs, NY: Prentice Hall, Inc.

Welsh, K. (2004). *African dance.* Philadelphia: Chelsea House Publishers.

Welsh Asante, K. (Ed.) (with quotes by Omofolabo Soyinka Ajayi and Felix Begho) (1996). *African dance: an artistic historical and philosophical inquiry.* African World Press, Inc.

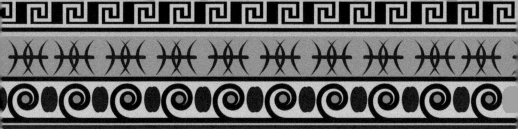

Chapter 5

FOUNDATIONS OF AFRICAN DANCE TECHNIQUES

U nlike other Western dances, African dances do not contain a common thread of dance movements. Each dance has its unique movements that tell a story. African dance utilizes the concept of polyrhythm, as well as total body articulation. Therefore, they relate to each other in the course of a dance performance. As stated in Chapter 3, African dance is about body isolations. This chapter will address these isolations and give you a sample of the techniques that are involved in executing the dances.

OVERVIEW OF AFRICAN DANCE MOVEMENTS

Several components of the body are isolated during African dance. These will be grouped as follows: legs and feet; arms, head, and neck; and torso and pelvis. The techniques for these four isolations will be discussed in this chapter. You will get a better understanding of African dance movements from these selected, step-by-step instructions. Small and large muscle groups are used in African dance.

Some terms associated with muscular and skeletal movements that need to be defined are:

1. **Protraction:** lengthening of the muscles
2. **Retraction:** shrinking of the muscles

3. **Supination:** a kind of rotation of the skeletal joints such as the arms and wrist, which allows the palm to be turned upward
4. **Pronation:** the act of rotating the arm so the palm is facing downward or backward
5. **Circumduction:** the circular movement of a limb

The following large and small muscle groups are used in the dance movements:

Techniques for Specific African Dances

As a student of African dance, you will have the opportunity to experience beginning and intermediate African dances. These dances are designed to give you an introduction to, as well as expose you to, dances that might have a difficulty level of low to medium. The dances taught in in the African Dance I class at George Mason University

Table 5.1 Muscle Groups Used in African Dance

UPPER BODY	
1. Chest	Pectoralis major
2. Upper/Middle Back	Trapezius/rhomboids (protraction & retraction)
3. Lower Back	Latissimus dorsi (protraction & retraction)
4. Shoulders	Anterior/posterior deltoids (rotation)
5. Arms	Biceps and triceps (supination & pronation)

MID-SECTION	
1. Stomach	Abdominals
2. Sides	Obliques

LOWER BODY	
1. Thighs	Quadriceps
2. Hamstrings	Biceps femoris
3. Buttocks	Gluteus maximus/medius (circumduction)
4. Hips/Pelvis	Iliopsoas (protraction & retraction)

are: **Djolo, Ma Gaue, Mystique, Koumbe Oleli, Cherie Nicaise, Somebody, Freedom, M'buta Zao, Dekonalan,** and **Fuba.** All of these dances were choreographed by Kukuwa Nuamah. This chapter describes some basic movements of each dance as it pertains to the legs and feet, the arms, and the torso and pelvis. For a comprehensive list of all the movements in these dances, refer to Chapter 6.

DJOLO

This dance is symbolic of a rite of passage. It depicts dancing into womanhood and manhood, and it is a dance of the West African countries of Ghana, Togo, Benin, and Ivory Coast. Initiation into adult life begins at an early age—nine for females and 13 for males. The initiates are schooled by the secrets and complexity of the older women and men in their communities. The men handle the boys as the women handle the girls. The choreography inspired by the song is taught in the African Dance I class. The basic dance movements of the legs and feet, the arms, and the torso of the first part of Djolo are described below. Complete movements of the dance are found in Chapter 6.

Leg and Foot Movement

Forward

The dance choreography is broken down in steps, starting with the right foot being tapped on the floor four times, followed by the left leg tapping on the floor for four counts.

> 1–4: Four steps forward, starting on the right foot, with elbows moving out and in on each step.
> 5–8: Four steps forward, starting on the left foot, with elbows moving out and in on each step.

Backward

Hands clap together above your head and then down behind the back, kicking legs forward, leaning backward with heel down and toes pointing up in the air for eight counts. One leg is always on floor while the other one is kicking in alternation.

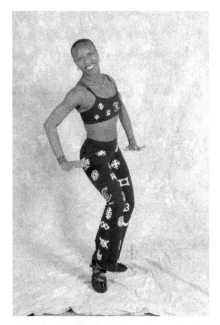

Figure 5.1 Forward Djolo leg movement.

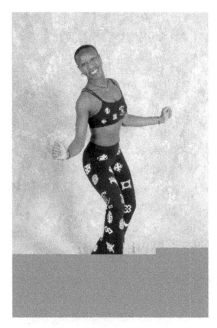

Figure 5.2 Backward Djolo leg movement.

Arms

Forward

Open hands, with palms directed up and out. Elbows are bent and move in toward the body and out.

Backward

Hands clap together above your head and then down behind your back.

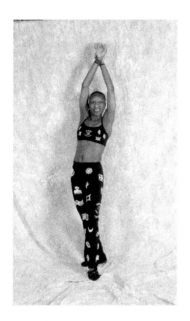

Figure **5.3** Forward Djolo arm movement.

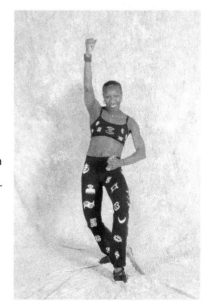

Figure **5.4** Backward Djolo arm movement.

Torso and Pelvis

Forward

The torso and pelvis are straight while tapping the feet.

Backward

The body leans back while you jump backward.

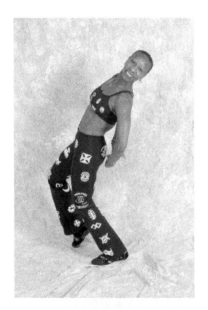

Figure 5.5 Forward Djolo torso and pelvic movement.

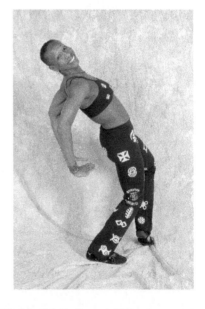

Figure 5.6 Backward Djolo torso and pelvic movement.

MA GAUE

Ma Gaue is a dance performed in West Africa to the ancestors as part of a birth ceremony. Births and ceremonies are taken very seriously by the African people, and each tribe performs its extensive rituals accordingly. The significance of this ceremony is the determination of how the child will fare in life. The choreography inspired by the song is taught in the African dance class. The basic dance movements of the legs and feet, the arms, and the torso of the first part of Ma Gaue are described below.

Leg and Foot Movement

Forward

Knees are in the bent position, then jump forward for four counts.

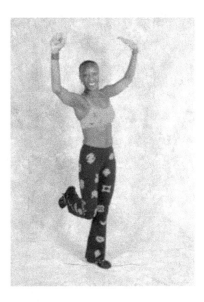

Figure 5.7 Forward Ma Gaue leg movement.

Backward

Jump backward four counts.

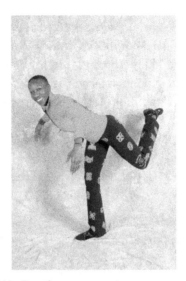

Figure 5.8 Backward Ma Gaue leg movement.

Arms

Forward

Begin with your arms straight up in the air, then shake your hands from side to side as your arms lower to the ground in between your legs.

Backward

Begin with your arms straight up in the air, then shake your hands from side to side as your arms lower to the ground in between your legs.

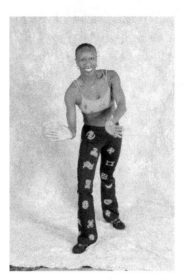

Figure 5.9 Forward Ma Gaue arm movement.

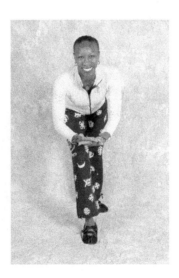

Figure 5.10 Backward Ma Gaue arm movement.

Torso and Pelvis

Forward

The pelvis tilts forward and back.

Backward

The pelvis tilts forward and back.

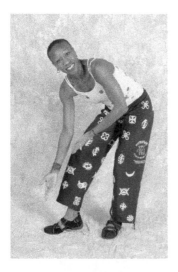

Figure 5.11 Forward Ma Gaue torso and pelvic movement.

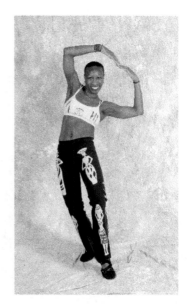

Figure 5.12 Backward Ma Gaue torso and pelvic movement.

MYSTIQUE

Mystique is a dance about the mysteries of the world. The world is a mystery to man, and in this dance, man takes different turns and avenues to figure out the intricacies of life. It is a Central African Dance performed by the people of Gabon, Cameroon, and the Democratic Republic of the Congo. The choreography inspired by the song is taught in the African Dance I class. The basic dance movements of the legs and feet, the arms, and the torso of the first part of Mystique are described below.

Leg and Foot Movement

Forward

Begin crouched down low to the ground with your knees bent.

1–8: Start with stepping back on your right foot while stepping forward with your left foot; then bring your right foot back together with your left foot. Now step back with your left foot while stepping forward with your right foot, and then bring your left foot back together with your right foot. You will alternate between starting with your right foot and left foot in eight counts.

Backward

1–4: Standing up straight, starting on the right, step back on one count.

5–8: Standing up straight, starting on the left, step backward on one count.

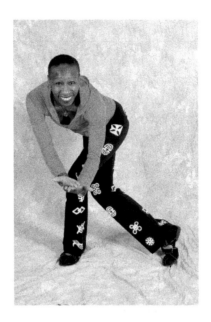

Figure 5.13 Forward Mystique leg movement.

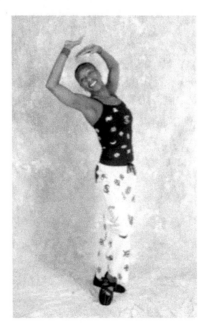

Figure 5.14 Backward Mystique leg movement.

Arms

Forward

9–16: As you move forward with your feet, move your arms, palms up, in an upward circular motion, over your head, around the sides of your body; then clasp your hands together the right hand inside of your left each time your arms pass your head. As your arms move, your head follows the direction of your arms. Repeat this circular movement with your arms while matching them to the steps of your feet.

Backward

Roll your hands in a circle in front of your head with your palms facing your face.

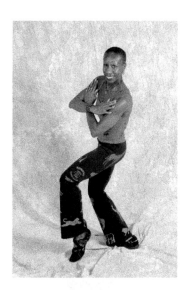

Figure 5.15 Forward Mystique arm movement.

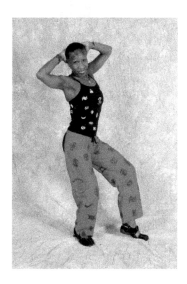

Figure 5.16 Backward Mystique arm movement.

Torso and Pelvis

Forward

The pelvis tilts forward and back.

Backward

The pelvis tilts forward and back.

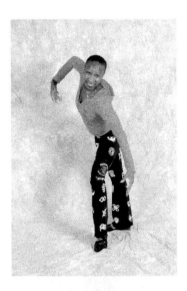

Figure 5.17 Forward Mystique torso and pelvic movement.

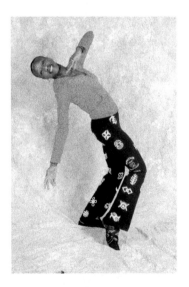

Figure 5.18 Backward Mystique torso and pelvic movement.

KOUMBE OLELI

Koumbe Oleli is a dance about warriors preparing for war and is performed by the West African people of Ghana. War is a manhood event for the Ashanti people; teenage boys are groomed and taught how to go to war to protect their people. The choreography inspired by the song is taught in the African Dance I class. The basic dance movements of the legs and feet, the arms, and the torso of the first part of Koumbe Oleli are described below.

Leg and Foot Movement

Forward

Right foot is tapped twice as it is shuffled forward. Left foot is then tapped twice as it is shuffled forward.

Backward

Right foot is tapped twice as it is shuffled backward. Left foot is then tapped twice as it is shuffled back.

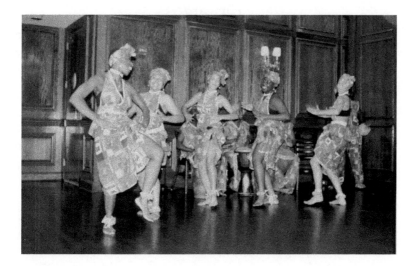

Figure 5.19 Forward Koumbe Oleli leg movement.

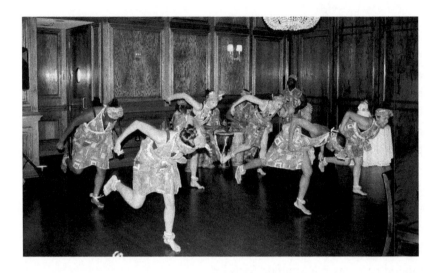

Figure 5.20 Backward Koumbe Oleli leg movement.

Arms

Forward

I–8: The elbows are bent and rolled forward one elbow at a time with the right one first, then the left one for eight counts toward the opponent as the body moves forward.

Backward

I–8: The elbows are bent and rolled backward, both elbows at the same time for eight counts away from the opponent as the body moves backward.

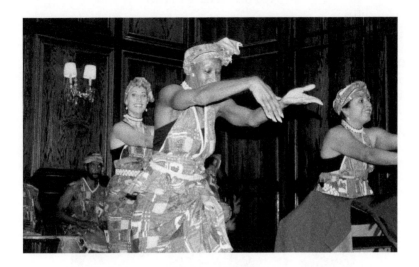

Figure 5.21 Forward Koumbe Oleli arm movement.

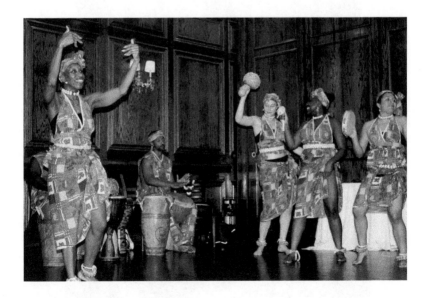

Figure 5.22 Backward Koumbe Oleli arm movement.

Torso and Pelvis

Forward

Torso is bent slightly forward.

Backward

Torso is bent slightly back.

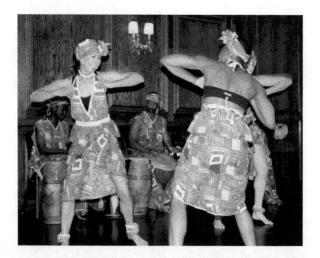

Figure 5.23 Forward Koumbe Oleli torso and pelvic movement.

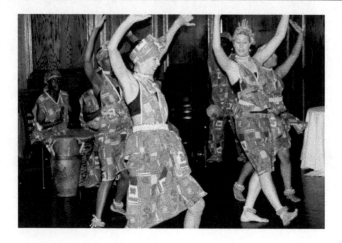

Figure 5.24 Backward Koumbe Oleli torso and pelvic movement.

CHERIE NICAISE

Cherie Nicaise is a dance performed by the central African countries of Cameroon and the Central African Republic. Beliefs and worship can get very deep for the tribes of Africa, and such dances are performed in reverence to both ancestors and other tribes for a pardon of a past wrong or for a request of a favor needed. The choreography inspired by the song is taught in the African Dance I class. The basic dance movements of the legs and feet, the arms, and the torso and pelvis of the first part of Cherie Nicaise are described below.

Leg and Foot Movement

Forward

The right foot is lifted and lowered, then the left foot.

Backward

1–8: Toes inward, knees inward and touching, as legs are turned inside and outside.

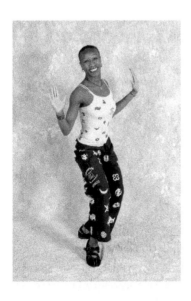

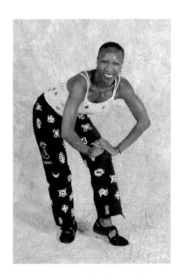

Figure 5.25 Forward Cherie Nicaise leg movement.

Figure 5.26 Backward Cherie Nicaise leg movement.

Arms

Forward

Move arms in a waving manner all the way upward toward the top of the head, clap, then down to the sides of the head for a count of four.

Backward

Arms are bent and kept close to the body and alternated inward and outward.

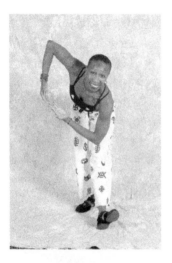

Figure 5.27 Forward Cherie Nicaise arm movement.

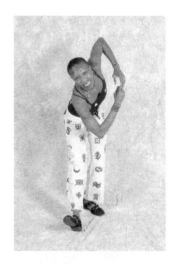

Figure 5.28 Backward Cherie Nicaise arm movement.

Torso and Pelvis

Forward

Hips are moved from side to side.

Backward

Torso is bent slightly back.

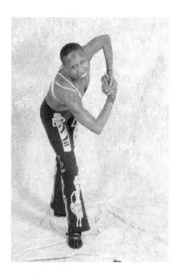

Figure 5.29 Forward Cherie Nicaise torso and pelvic movement.

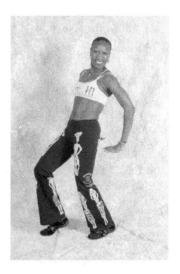

Figure 5.30 Backward Cherie Nicaise torso and pelvic movement.

SOMEBODY

Somebody is a dance that is representative of the type of choreography currently originating in Africa. It is an example of an original contemporary dance. "Somebody" is a song that originated during the apartheid era, when the people of South Africa went through oppression and hard times. Knocks on the doors were so frightening and uncertain during those times that no one answered their doors, but rather took cover to protect their lives. Choreography was inspired by the song "Somebody," and the basic dance movements of the legs and feet, the arms, and the torso and pelvis of the first part of the choreography are described below.

Leg and Foot Movement

Forward

1–8: The feet are apart and moving in a single, single, double, double, motion for eight counts.

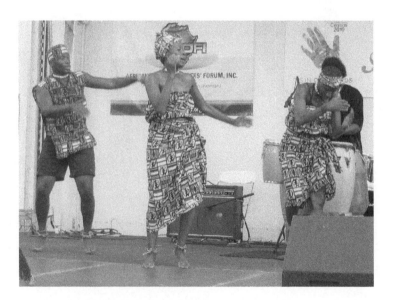

Figure 5.31 Forward Somebody leg movement.

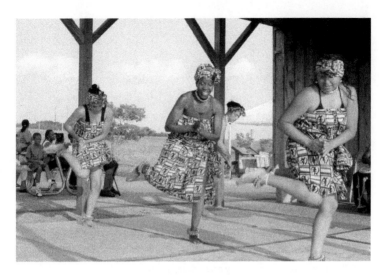

Figure 5.32 Backward Somebody leg movement.

Arms

Forward

Hands in a fist in a double motion.

9–16: Hands clasped behind the head and elbows out to the right and left.

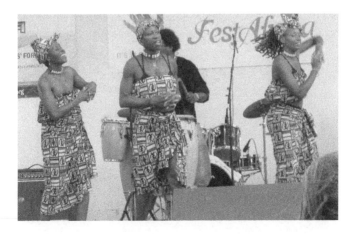

Figure 5.33 Forward Somebody arm movement.

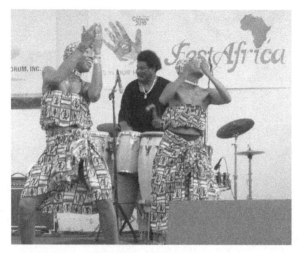

Figure 5.34 Backward Somebody arm movement.

Torso and Pelvis

Forward

Torso is straight.

Backward

Body bent low toward the ground and moving backward in eight counts.

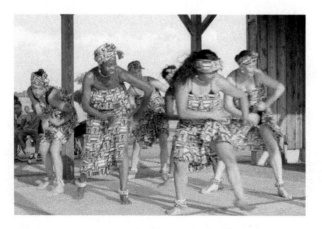

Figure 5.35 Forward Somebody torso and pelvic movement.

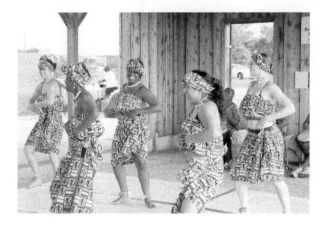

Figure 5.36 Backward Somebody torso and pelvic movement.

FREEDOM

Freedom is an example of a dance that tells the story of something that happened in Africa. These kinds of dances have been performed in Africa for centuries, originally depicting ancient myths. However, Freedom is much more recent. During the era of apartheid, the South Africans were ruled with an iron fist by their oppressors, the Europeans. They were tortured, whipped, imprisoned, battered, and killed. Eventually, they won their freedom, and their hero, the late Nelson Mandela, the leader of the African National Congress, was freed after 27 years of imprisonment. This Zulu dance signifies the bondage before and exemplifies the freedom they have now attained. The basic dance movements of the legs and feet, the arms, and the torso and pelvis of the first part of the choreography are described below.

Leg and Foot Movement

Forward

Starting with the right foot tapping on the floor two times, bring the knees up high, followed by the left leg tapping on the floor for two counts.

Backward

Starting with the right foot tapping on the floor two times, bring the knees up high, followed by the left leg tapping on the floor, also two counts.

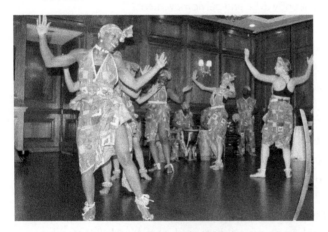

Figure 5.37 Forward Freedom leg movement.

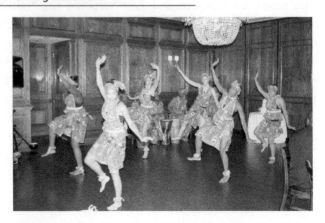

Figure 5.38 Backward Freedom leg movement.

Arms

Forward

Start with your arms straight up, then roll your hands from side to side as your arms lower to the ground in between your legs; your head follows your arms. Repeat this for four counts.

Backward

Extend arms out backward, then up and over the right shoulder. Extend arms out backward, then up and over the left shoulder.

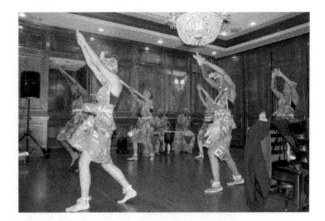

Figure 5.39 Forward Freedom arm movement.

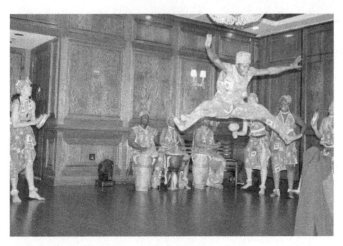

Figure 5.40 Backward Freedom arm movement.

Torso and Pelvis

Forward

Jump forward one step; pelvis moves tilting forward and back.

Backward

Torso is bent forward.

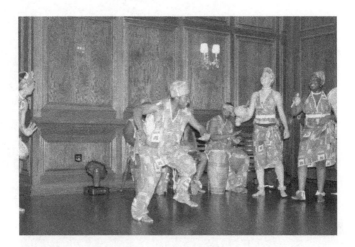

Figure 5.41 Forward Freedom torso and pelvic movement.

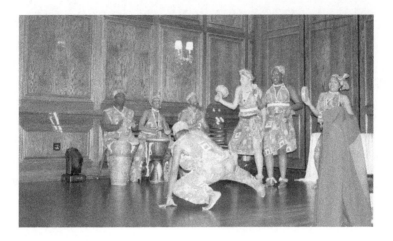

Figure 5.42 Backward Freedom torso and pelvic movement.

M'BUTA ZAO

M'buta Zao is a dance originating from central Africa, specifically, Cameroon and the Republic of the Congo. Power and loyalty are symbolized in this dance. African men are the heads of their families and possess the power to be in charge of the household in caring and feeding the household members. This sort of power allows the women the respect for their men. In return, the women play their roles in loyalty and obedience to their men. The choreography inspired by the song is taught in the African Dance I class. The basic dance movements of the legs and feet, arms, and the torso and pelvis of the first part of the choreography are described below.

Leg and Foot Movement

Forward

Step back, alternating the left and right feet for eight counts.

Backward

Step back, double count left and right.

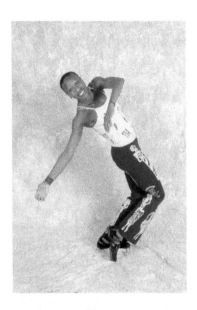

Figure **5.43** Forward M'buta Zao leg movement.

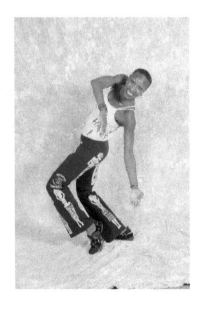

Figure **5.44** Backward M'buta Zao leg movement.

Arms

Forward

Both arms are swaying sideways; first the right side, then the left side.

Backward

The hands are behind the middle back, with the right hand into the left hand.

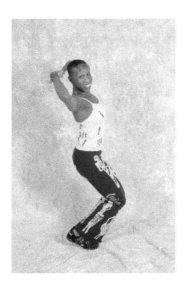

Figure 5.45 Forward M'buta Zao arm movement.

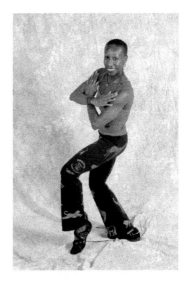

Figure 5.46 Backward M'buta Zao arm movement.

Torso and Pelvis

Forward

The shoulders jerk forward and backward for eight counts.

Backward

The body moves lower in a forward motion.

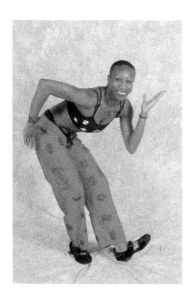

Figure 5.47 Forward M'buta Zao torso and pelvic movement.

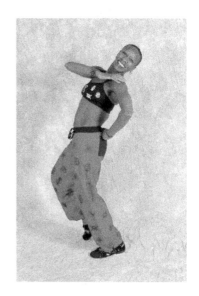

Figure 5.48 Backward M'buta Zao torso and pelvic movement.

DEKONALAN

Dekonalan is a dance that pertains to the West African people, specifically the people of Togo and Benin. Ceremonies are performed during the time of seed sowing for the villages and townships in order for blessings to be received for their harvests. These dances are performed in respect to their ancestors, whom they believe have a much better connection to Mother Earth. The choreography inspired by the ceremonial dances is taught in the African Dance I class. The basic dance movements of the legs and feet, arms, and the torso and pelvis of the first part of the choreography are described below.

Leg and Foot Movement

Forward

This dance begins with the right heel and toe twisting into the ground for four counts.

It then switches to the left heel and toe twisting into the ground for four counts.

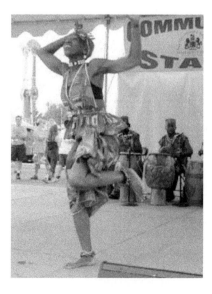

Figure 5.49 Forward Dekonalan leg movement.

Backward

Hop backward on heel alone on right foot, then on left foot.

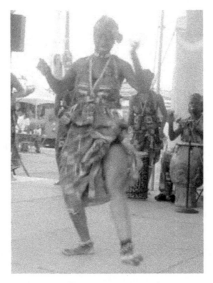

Figure 5.50 Backward Dekonalan leg movement.

Arms

Forward

The hands are twisted back and forth, synchronized with the feet for four counts.

Backward

Sway both arms to the right, then to the left.

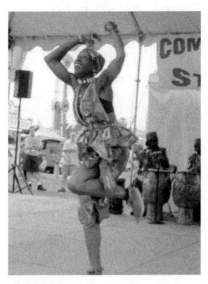

Figure 5.51 Forward Dekonalan arm movement.

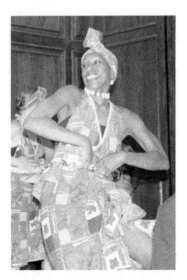

Figure 5.52 Backward Dekonalan arm movement.

Torso and Pelvis

Forward

Pelvis twists with arm and leg movement.

Backward

Wiggle the body left and right.

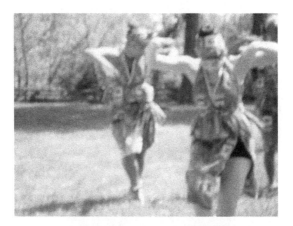

Figure 5.53 Forward Dekonalan torso and pelvic movement.

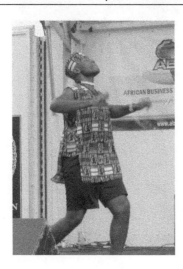

Figure 5.54 Backward Dekonalan torso and pelvic movement.

FUBA

Fuba is a dance indicative of the rain dance of Northern Ghana and Burkina Faso. Rain can be very scarce in Africa at times. There are two seasons in sub-Saharan Africa: the rainy season and the dry season. Just about at the end of the dry season, the tribes perform several tribal rain dances to their ancestors in a plea for rain from the heavens for their crops and daily lives. The choreography inspired by the rain dances is taught in the African Dance I class. The basic dance movements of the legs and feet, arms, and the torso and pelvis of the first part of the choreography are described below.

Leg and Foot Movement

Forward

Right, left, right, right, right.

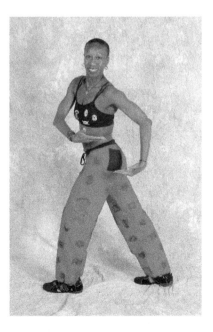

Figure 5.55 Forward Fuba leg movement.

Backward

Left, right, left, left, left.

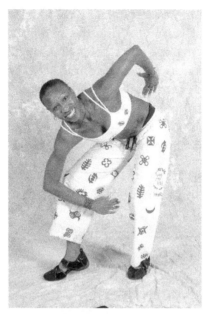

Figure 5.56 Backward Fuba movement.

Arms

Forward

Starting from below with legs apart and clapping in between the legs, then up above heads.

Immediately after the claps, begin moving forward in a fast rhythmic drum movement, with hands rubbing against each other downward, then upward for eight counts.

Backward

Do the same movement backward, but rub your hands downward, then to the right, and then again downward, then to the left for eight counts backward.

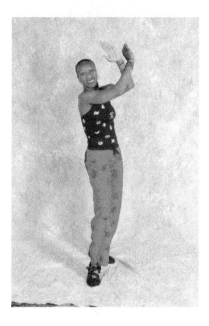

Figure 5.57 Forward Fuba arm movement.

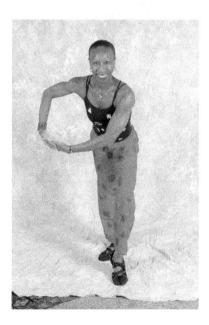

Figure 5.58 Backward Fuba arm movement.

Torso and Pelvis

Forward

Bent and straightened.

Backward

Bent and straightened.

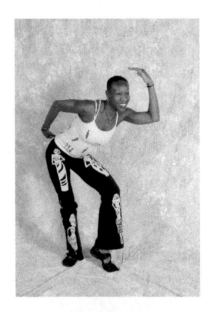

Figure 5.59 Forward Fuba torso and pelvic movement.

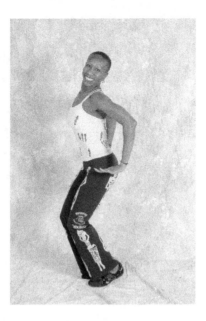

Figure 5.60 Backward Fuba torso and pelvic movement.

SUMMARY

The ten dances listed for the African Dance I classes cover a range of ceremonial, beliefs, and ritualistic dancing. Some of the dances taught incorporate the actual dance movements of the regions, while others are dances inspired by the message of the songs. In all, the authentic African movement is evident. Both beginning and intermediate dances are incorporated into the African Dance I class. Students will emerge from this class with a better understanding and proper execution of the dance movements. This chapter introduces the beginning movements of these dances. Complete descriptions of all of the movements within these dances are discussed in Chapter 6.

GLOSSARY

Cherie Nicaise	A beliefs and worship dance performed in reverence to both ancestors and other tribes for a pardon of something done wrong, or for a request of a favor needed
Circumduction	The circular movement of a limb
Dekonalan	A ceremonial dance performed during the time of seed sowing for the villages and townships in order for blessings to be received for their harvests.
Djolo	A West African Dance into man- and womanhood
Freedom	A Zulu dance that signifies the bondage of the South Africans and their ensuing freedom
Fuba	Several tribal rain dances performed to their God, so He may send down rain from above for their physical needs and everyday lives
Koumbe Oleli	A dance about warriors preparing for war that is performed by the West African people of Ghana, the Ashanti tribe
Ma Gaue	A births and ceremonies dance from West Africa performed to their ancestors
M'buta Zao	A power and loyalty dance that originates from Cameroon and the Republic of Congo
Mystique	A central African dance about the mysteries of life
Pronation	The act of rotating the arm so the palm is facing downward or backward
Protraction	The lengthening of the muscles
Retraction	The shrinking of the muscles
Somebody	A dance originated during the apartheid era, when the people of South Africa went through oppression and hard times.
Supination	A kind of rotation of the skeletal joints such as the arms and wrist, which allows the palm to be turned upward.

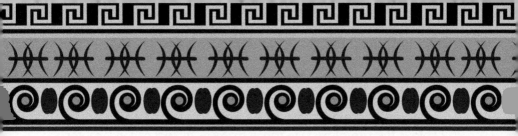

Chapter 6

Template for African Dances Taught in Class

I n your African dance classes, you will learn various African dances that entail unique movements that tell a story. Chapter 5 introduced body movements of the legs and feet, the arms, and the torso and pelvis of the dances presented. In this chapter, the ten dances introduced in Chapter 5 are presented in their entirety from beginning to end. The dances described are: **Djolo**, **Ma Gaue**, **Mystique**, **Koumbe Oleli**, **Cherie Nicaise**, **Somebody**, **Freedom**, **M'buta Zao**, **Dekonalan**, and **Fuba**. These dances are listed in the order they are taught in African Dance 1 class at George Mason University. It's worth mentioning that while some of these dances bear some of the historical and cultural dances of the countries presented, others are original choreography using African dance moves to portray the story being told.

DJOLO

Djolo is the rite-of-passage dance that was introduced in Chapter 5.

Dance Formation

Body facing

Face the front of the class to begin with and perform movements forward and backward, as well as side to side. The first rule in African dance: When the arms move in a direction, the head follows in that same direction. The second rule is that the majority of the movements are with bent knee so the dancer is lower to the ground. The third rule is that the right hand is the respectful hand in the African culture; therefore, we give that respect to starting all dances on the right.

Music

Each dance has its own specific music written and played by the artists, but as with African dances, the drummers play for the dancers to perform, so the music used for the dances is usually drumming. A story of the dance is told as a lecture, then the choreography of the dance is taught in steps.

Section A

Forward

Starting body position: The dance choreography is broken down in steps, starting with the right foot tapping on the floor four times, followed by the left leg tapping on the floor also for four counts. (Not the same for all the dances, some have to start with the arms and the head first.)

Open hands, with palms directed up and out, elbows move out first, then in second. If you move your elbow out and in, your four-count feet movement will fall in count with it.

1–4: Four steps forward, starting on the right foot, with elbows moving out and in on each step.

5–8: Four steps forward, starting on the left foot, with elbows moving out and in on each step.

Backward

Body leans back while doing a leaning-back jumping jack. Hands clasp together above your head and then down behind the back, kicking legs forward, leaning back with heel down and toes pointing up in the air for eight counts. One leg is always on floor, while the other one is kicking in alternation.

Section B

Forward

1–4: Head facing forward, body facing forward, arms bent at elbow, hands in fists and held out beside the body. The body is facing forward, while the pelvis is tilted forward and back and the head is also up and down in four counts. The fists move in the direction of the arms.

5–8: Standing in place for each four-count before moving on to the next count and moving pelvis. In all the dances, pelvic movement is key and is always moved in a tilting position forward and backward.

Forward

Move forward toward the front of the studio:

1. Right step forward, pelvic moves tilting forward and backward, arms bent at elbow and out to side of body, head up.

2. Left step forward, pelvic moves, tilting forward and backward arms bent at elbow and into side of body, head down.

3. Right step forward, pelvic moves, tilting forward and backward, arms bent at elbow and out to side of body, head up.
4. Left step forward, pelvic moves, tilting forward and backward, arms bent at elbow and into side of body, head down,

Repeat four counts, starting with the right foot.

Backward

Move backward to the back of the studio, right side of the studio to the left side of the studio, moving backward for eight counts.

1. Right step backward, pelvic moves tilting forward and backward, arms bent at elbow and out to side of body, head up.
2. Left step backward, pelvic moves tilting forward and backward, arms bent at elbow and into side of body, head down.
3. Right step backward, pelvic moves tilting forward and backward, arms bent at elbow and out to side of body, head up.
4. Left step backward, pelvic moves tilting forward and backward, arms bent at elbow and into side of body, head down.

Repeat four counts, starting with the right foot.
When the head is up or down, the face focuses on the ceiling for up and the floor for down.

Section C

Forward

Body position: slightly bending forward, put your right hand on top of your left hand with both palms open.

1–4: Circling upward right to straight (aligned) position, the head follows the body movement, and the dancer is moving her body to the side as she circles up.

5–8: Circling downward left and down to bent knee position, head follows the body movement, and dancer is moving her body to the side as she circles up.

Backward

1–4: Standing up straight, starting on the right, step backward on two counts, put your hands on your stomach, and shrug your elbows backward.

5–8: Standing up straight, starting on the left, step backward, on two counts, put your hands on your stomach, and shrug your elbows backward.

Section D

Jumping with arms out.

Body position is turned facing toward the right-hand side of the room.

Right arm "out and up," stretched out to the side of the body.

1–4: Jump from both feet to right foot, placing feet flat on floor, right arm out and up, left arm out and down, head follows right arm up. The arm movements occur throughout the four counts, with four hops to the right.

5–8: Jump from both feet to left foot, placing feet flat on floor, left arm out and up, right arm out and down, head follows left arm up. The arm movements occur throughout the four counts, with four hops to the left.

Repeat four counts, starting with the right foot.

Section E

Circling, jiggle stomach.

(This step may be challenging at first for students, but with practice it becomes easier.).

1–4: Four steps to the right, pelvis moves forward and back in a fast motion, jiggle stomach while circling open hands to the right.

The palms face the outside away from the body, and the circling is complete round circles to the right, then to the left.

5–8: Four steps to the right, pelvis moves forward and back in a fast motion, jiggle stomach while circling open hands to the right.

The palms face the outside away from the body, and the circling is complete round circles to the left, then to the right.

Ma Gaue

Ma Gaue is the birth ceremony dance introduced in Chapter 5.

Section A

Starting body position: Begin with your knees bent and your arms straight up with your hands in a clawlike position, as if holding a baby up to the skies.

Forward

Move forward toward the front of the studio.

1–4: With your arms straight up, jump forward one step, pelvic moves tilting forward and backward, then roll your hands from side to side as your arms lower to the ground in between your legs; your head follows your arms; repeat this for four counts.

Backward

Move backward toward the back of the studio.

5–8: With your arms straight up, jump backward one step, pelvic moves tilting forward and backward, then roll your hands from side to side as your arms lower to the ground in between your legs; your head follows your arms; repeat this for four counts.

Section B

Forward

Move forward toward the front of the studio.

1–8: Crouch down low with your knees bent, place your right hand in front of your left hand with your palms facing you, pelvis moves tilting forward and backward, arms bent at elbow and into the side of the body, head down, rotate your elbows inward and outward as you take one step in front of the other for eight steps.

Backward

Move backward toward the back of the studio.

9–16: With your knees still bent, fold your thumbs into your hands to make two fists. Lean to the left, pelvic moves tilting forward and backward, roll your fist inward toward you four times, then clap. Lean to the left, pelvic moves tilting forward and backward, roll your fist inward toward you four times, then clap. Alternate between right and left for eight counts.

Section C

Forward

Right side of the studio to the left side of the studio.

1–4: Weave your fingers together and then place them behind your head, elbows bent and sticking out; rotate your right ankle inward while poking your left hip outward, then slide your right ankle and hip outward. Move your head in the same direction your ankle is facing. Move toward the right side of the studio for four counts.

Backward

Left side of the studio to the right side of the studio.

5–8: Turn your body to the left side of the studio, rotate your left ankle inward while poking your right hip outward, then slide your left ankle and hip outward. Move your head in the same direction your ankle is facing. Move toward the left side of the studio for four counts.

Section D

Forward

Move forward toward the front of the studio:

1. Begin standing with your knees slightly bent, step out with your right foot, rotate your right ankle outward, extend your arms out to your right side, and let them sway as your right ankle rotates inward and outward for four counts.
2. Step out with your left foot, rotate your left ankle outward, extend your arms out to your left side, and let them sway as your left ankle rotates inward and outward for four counts.
3. Step out with your right foot, rotate your right ankle outward, extend your arms out to your right side, and let them sway as your right ankle rotates inward and outward for four counts.
4. Step out with your left foot, rotate your left ankle outward, extend your arms out to your left side, and let them sway as your left ankle rotates inward and outward for four counts.

Backward

Move backward toward the back of the studio.

1–8: Clasp your fingers tightly together and extend them up and out over the right side of your head; roll your hands three times outward as you run backward toward the back of the studio. Then bring your hands down to the left side of your leg and roll them outward three times. You will alternate between rolling your hands on the right and left side of you as your run backward for eight counts and end on the right knee, with your right hand in your left hand on the floor.

CHERIE NICAISE

Cherie Nicaise is the beliefs and worship dance that was introduced in Chapter 5.

Section A

Starting body position is hips moving side to side and arms clapping above the head.

Forward

1–4: Move the body side to side from the hips including butt (boombsey), making sure the butt is actually moving more than the hips.

5–8: Move arms in a waving manner all the way up toward the top of the head, clap, then down to the sides of the head, in a count of four.

Repeat this four times moving forward.

Backward

1–8 Toes inward, knees inward and touching as legs are turned inside and outside. Head forward and downward, then upward and backward, hands held very close to the body.

Section B

Sideways

1–4: Move body toward the right side four counts on a down/up step movement, then move body toward the left side four counts on a down/up step movement.

5–8: Roll hands toward the face as you move side to side on four counts to right and left.

Section C

Forward

1–4: Stretch right arm outward with hand out, then stretch left hand outward with hand out under right hand, and begin to turn counterclockwise for four counts.

5–8: Stretch left arm outward with hand out, then stretch right hand outward with hand out over left hand, and begin to turn clockwise for four counts.

Backward

1–8: Move body forward and backward toward the back with toes inward, knees inward and touching as legs are turned inside and outside for eight counts backward.

MYSTIQUE

Mystique is the mysteries of life dance introduced in Chapter 5.

Section A

Starting body position: Begin crouched down low to the ground with your knees bent.

Forward

1–8: Start with stepping back on your right foot while stepping forward with your left foot, and then bring your right foot back together with your left foot. Then step back with your left foot while stepping forward with your right foot, and then bring your left foot back together with your right foot. Alternate between starting with your right foot and left foot in eight counts.

9–16: As you move forward with your feet, move your arms, palms up, in an upward circular motion over your head, around the sides of your body, and then clasp your hands together, right hand inside of your left each time your arms pass your head. As your arms move, your head follows the direction of your arms. Repeat this circular movement with your arms while matching them to the steps of your feet.

Backward

1–4: Standing up straight, starting on the right, step backward on one count, pelvic moves tilting forward and backward, then roll your hands in a circle in front of your head with your palms facing your face.

5–8: Standing up straight, starting on the left, step backward on one count, pelvic moves tilting forward and backward, then roll your hands in a circle in front of your head with your palms facing your face.

Section B

Forward

1–4: Four steps forward, pelvis moves forward and backward in a fast motion, extend your right arm as you step your right foot, then extend your left arm as you step your left foot. Next, bring your right hand to your left shoulder as you step with your right foot again, and then bring your left hand to your right shoulder as you step with your left foot again, giving the appearance of your arms crossed around your chest. Finally, turn counterclockwise in a full circle while moving your pelvis forward and backward in a rigorous manner.

Backward

1–4: Standing up straight, starting on the right, step backward on one count, pelvic moves tilting forward and backward; then roll your hands in a circle in front of your head with your palms facing your face.

5–8: Standing up straight, starting on the left, step backward on one count, pelvic moves tilting forward and backward; then roll your hands in a circle in front of your head with your palms facing your face.

Section C

Forward

1–4: Four steps forward, pelvis moves forward and backward in a fast motion, extend your right arm as you step your right foot, then extend your left arm as you step your left foot. Next, bring your right hand to the right backside of your head as you step with your right foot again, and then bring your left hand to the left backside of your head as you step with your left foot again; lace your fingers behind your head. Finally, turn counterclockwise in a full circle while moving your pelvis forward and back in a rigorous manner.

Backward

1–4: Standing up straight, starting on the right, step backward on one count, pelvic moves tilting forward and backward; then roll your hands in a circle in front of your head with your palms facing your face.

5–8: Standing up straight, starting on the left, step backward on one count, pelvic moves tilting forward and backward; then roll your hands in a circle in front of your head with your palms facing your face.

Section D

Body position is turned facing toward the right-hand side of room.
Right arm "out and up," stretched out to the side of the body.

1–4: Raise right arm and foot out and up, left arm extended out in front of the body with palm facing outward; head follows right arm up. The arm movements occur throughout the four counts, with four hops to the right.

5–8: Raise left arm and foot out and up, right arm extended out in front of the body with palm facing outward; head follows left arm up. The arm movements occur throughout the four counts, with four hops to the left.

Repeat four counts starting with the right foot.

Section E

Counterclockwise

1. Move your right arm over your shoulder, pushing down the air in front of you; let your head follow your arm as it moves over your right shoulder. Lift your right foot up and back as your right arm moves and then back to the ground when your arm moves in front of you.
2. Move your left arm over your shoulder, pushing down the air in front of you; let your head follow your arm as it moves over your left shoulder. Lift your left foot up and back as your left arm moves and then back to the ground when your arm moves in front of you.
3. Alternate between your left and right arm for eight counts, turning counterclockwise in a circle.

Clockwise

1. Move your right arm over your shoulder, pushing down the air in front of you; let your head follow your arm as it moves over your right shoulder. Lift your right foot up and back as your right arm moves and then back to the ground when your arm moves in front of you.
2. Move your left arm over your shoulder, pushing down the air in front of you; let your head follow your arm as it moves over your left shoulder. Lift your left foot up and back as your left arm moves and then back to the ground when your arm moves in front of you.
3. Alternate between your left and right arm for 8 counts turning clockwise in a circle.

KOUMBE OLELI

Koumbe Oleli is a dance about warriors preparing for war and is performed by the West African people of Ghana. War is a manhood event for the Ashanti people. In a boy's teen years, he is groomed and taught how to go to war to protect his community.

Starting body position: This dance starts with the body in a bending-forward position as two dance groups face each other as in preparation for war. The arms are also bent at the elbows and the hands are in fist position, resting on the shoulders.

Both dance groups yell out loud sounds like grunts and shouts to intimidate the opponent as they get closer in toward each other.

Section A

Forward

1–8: The elbows are rolling forward one elbow at a time, with right one first, then the left one for eight counts toward the opponent as the body moves forward.

Backward

1–8: The elbows still in the same position are now both rolling backward for eight counts as the body moves backward along with the counts.

Both dance groups yell out loud sounds like grunts and shouts to intimidate the opponent as they get closer to each other.

Section B

Forward

1–8: The arms are now stretched upward toward the skies in two counts and then lowered straight down toward the ground in two counts. The body moves forward for eight counts with this move toward the opponent again.

Backward

9–16: The arms stretched out upward and downward, still in two counts, with the body moving backward, this time for eight counts.

Both dance groups yell out loud grunts and shouts to intimidate the opponent as they get closer to each other.

Section C

Forward

1–8: The arms are now stretched open completely to the side of the body, then brought together for a loud clap to the front of the body as the body moves forward and inward toward the opponent.

Facing each other:

The two dance groups (opponents) facing each other now stretch out their arms in reach of each other's arms as they leap off their feet in dance with head moving up and down, along with arm movements.

1–16: They reach out for 16 counts, and on the last count, they kneel down on the right knee with arms still touching and stretched out.

SOMEBODY

Somebody is the contemporary dance we encountered in Chapter 5.

Starting body position: Both hands are in a fist position (thumb down and fingers covering thumb) above the head and pretend knocking on the door.

Section A

Forward

1–8: The feet are apart and moving in a single, single, double, double motion for eight counts.

Backward

9–16: Hands clasped behind the head, elbows out to the right and left. Body bent low toward the ground and moving backward in eight counts.

Section B

1–8: Toes inward, knees inward and touching as legs are turned inside and outside. Head forward and downward, then upward and backward; hands held in front of body.

Counterclockwise

1. Move body forward and backward in the position above for four counts at each angle around the room counterclockwise.
2. Move the body in the motion with arms stretched out and hands touching at the tips of the fingers as in a cat-and-mouse chase (catch and release).

Clockwise

1. Move body forward and backward in the position above for four counts at each angle around the room clockwise
2. Move the body in the motion with arms stretched out and hands touching at the tips of the fingers as in a cat-and-mouse chase (catch and release).

Section C

Forward

1–8: Running away from oppressors: the body is bent over low in a running position with runner hands on sides of the body and head facing left for two counts and then right for two counts in a running motion.

Backward

9–16: Pulling away from oppressors when caught, body is bent at the knee lower to the ground and arms are in a pulling position.

Right arm pulls as left arm stretches, then alternate, so the left arm pulls as the right arm stretches for two counts each.

FREEDOM

Freedom is the storytelling dance that was introduced in Chapter 5.

Section A

Starting body position: Begin with your knees bent and your arms straight up with your hands in a clawlike position, as if you're trying to grab something.

Forward

Move forward toward the front of the studio.

1–4: With your arms straight up, jump forward one step, pelvic moves tilting forward and backward, then roll your hands from side to side as your arms lower toward the ground in between your legs; your head follows your arms; repeat this for four counts.

Backward:

Move backward toward back of studio.

Start with the right foot tapping on the floor two times; bring the knees up high, followed by the left leg tapping on the floor, also two counts.

1–4: 4 Step forward, starting on the right foot, extend arms out backward, then up and over the right shoulder as you tap your feet on the ground; bring your knees up high each time you step.

5–8: 4 Step forward, starting on the right foot, extend arms out backward, then up and over the left shoulder as you tap your feet on the ground; bring your knees up high each time you step.

Section B

Forward

Counterclockwise in a circle.

1. Crouch down low with your knees bent; fold your thumbs inside your hands to make two fists. Jump in place as your cross your arms and legs, then uncross them, then recross them again, this time getting as low to the ground as you can. Make sure to jump every time you cross and uncross your arms and legs. Every time your arms are crossed, your head should be facing down; every time your arms and legs are uncrossed, your head should be facing up.
2. Jump in place as you uncross your arms and legs, then cross them, then uncross them again, this time with your knees bent and your feet firmly placed on the ground, elbows bent, fingers spaced out with palms facing away from you. Yell "Hey!" as you throw your head back.

Then turn to your left for three counts and repeat until you are facing the front of the studio again.

Backward

Clockwise in a circle.

1. Turn to the right, cross your arms and legs, then uncross them, then recross them again, this time getting as low to the ground as you can. Make sure to jump every time you cross and uncross your arms and legs.
2. Jump in place as you uncross your arms and legs, then cross them, then uncross them again, this time with your knees bent and your feet firmly placed on the ground, elbows bent, fingers spaced out with palms facing away from you. Yell "Hey!" as you throw your head back.

Then turn to your right and repeat for two more counts.

Section C

Forward

Move forward to the front of the studio.

1–4: Four steps forward, starting on the right foot; raise your right foot back and out, then return it to the ground two times; fold your thumbs in your right hand to make a fist, extend arms up and over the right side, then bring your right fist down toward your shoulder two times. Move your head along with your hand.

5–8: Four steps forward, starting on the left foot, raise your left foot back and out, then return it to the ground two times. Fold your thumb in your left hand to make a fist, extend arms up and over the left side, then bring your left fist down toward your shoulder two times. Move your head along with your hand.

Backward

Move backward toward the back of the studio.

Starting with the right foot tapping on the floor two times, followed by the left leg tapping on the floor, also two counts.

1–4: Four steps forward, starting on the right foot, bringing the knees up high, fists together, with elbows moving up and down on each step.

5–8: Four steps forward, starting on the left foot, keeping the knees up high, fists together, with elbows moving up and down on each step.

M'BUTA ZAO

M'buta Zao is the loyalty dance we learned about in Chapter 5.

Section A

This dance is divided into two parts—the male part and the female part—but the two are combined during the dance. (This dance can be performed by both males and females alike.)

Forward

1–8: The first female part begins this dance with the body moving low in forward motion, with legs stepping backward like a pachanga step for eight counts. Both arms are swaying sideways, first the right side, then the left side.

Backward

9–16: The female part continues with the hands behind the middle back, with the right hand into the left hand and the shoulders jerking forward and backward, moving the body for eight counts.

Section B

Forward counterclockwise:

1. The man's part is inserted right here with the arms in four strong positions. The first position of the arms is fisted with elbows out to the right and left, with fists resting on the chest while elbows rotate backward, with a jump forward.
2. The second position of the arms is to stretch out both arms, right and left, straight out, with hands fisted at the end while the arms rotate backward, with a jump forward and to the left.
3. The third position of the arms is to have both arms bent, also fisted, behind the head while the arms rotate backward (hard to do), with a jump forward and toward the left.

4. The fourth position of the arms is to have both arms bent behind the body, fisted right into the lower back, with a last jump forward toward the left.

Backward clockwise:

5. The man's part is inserted right here, again with the arms in four strong positions. The first position of the arms is fisted with elbows out to the right and left, with fists resting on the chest while elbows rotate backward, with a jump forward.
6. The second position of the arms is to stretch out both arms right and left, straight out, with hands fisted at the end while arms rotate backward, with a jump forward and toward the right.
7. The third position of the arms is to have both arms bent, also fisted, behind the head while the arms rotate backward (hard to do), with a jump forward and to the right.
8. The fourth position of the arms is to have both arms bent behind the body, fisted right into the lower back, with a last jump forward toward the right.

Forward

1–8: The second female part begins this dance with the body moving low in forward motion, with the arms touching shoulders crisscross, and then touching thighs, also crisscross.
The legs are backward steps like a pachanga step for eight counts.

Backward

9–16: The female part continues with the hands behind the middle back, with the right hand into the left hand and the shoulders jerking forward and backward, with body movements for eight counts.

Section C

Forward counterclockwise

1. The man's part is inserted once again right here, with the arms in four strong positions. The first position of the arms is fisted, with elbows out to the right and left, with fists resting on the chest while the elbows rotate backward with a jump forward.

2. The second position of the arms is to stretch out both arms, right and left, straight out, with hands fisted at the end while the arms rotate backward with a jump forward and toward the left.

3. The third position of the arms is to have both arms, also fisted, bent behind the head while the arms rotate backward (hard to do), with a jump forward and toward the left.

4. The fourth position of the arms is to have both arms, also fisted, bent behind the body, fisted right into the lower back, with a last jump forward toward the left.

Backward clockwise

5. The man's part is inserted here, again with the arms in four strong positions. The first position of the arms is fisted with elbows out to the right and left, with fists resting on the chest while elbows rotate backward, with a jump forward.

6. The second position of the arms is to stretch out both arms, right and left, straight out, with hands fisted at the end while arms rotate backward, with a jump forward and toward the right.

7. The third position of the arms is to have both arms fisted and bent behind the head while the arms rotate backward (hard to do), with a jump forward and toward the right.

8. The fourth position of the arms is to have both arms fisted and bent behind the body, fisted right into the lower back, with a last jump forward toward the right to finish the dance.

DEKONALAN

Dekonalan is the harvest dance introduced in Chapter 5.

Section A

Forward

1–4: This dance begins with the right heel and toe twisting into the ground for four counts. The hands also twist back and forth in sync with the feet for four counts.

5–8: Switch to the left heel and toe, twisting into the ground for four counts. The hands also twist back and forth in sync with the feet for four counts.

Repeat the above moves for another four counts on each foot.

Backward

1–8: Hop backward on heel alone on right foot, then on left foot, and sway arms to the right and then to the left, shaking and wiggling the body at same time.

Section B

Counterclockwise

1. Move right heel and toe in twisting motion again and move counterclockwise for eight counts, with arms flapping close to body.

Clockwise

2. Move left heel and toe in twisting motion again and move clockwise for eight counts, with arms flapping close to body.

Section C

Forward

1–8: Begin by touching the ground with your hands, palms down as in planting seeds. Bend knees and move in a down-and-up motion with your body as you touch the ground; raise up and touch again for eight counts moving parallel forward.

Backward

9–16: Begin by touching the ground with your hands, palms down as in planting seeds. Bend knees and move in a down-and-up motion with your body as you touch the ground; raise up and touch again for eight counts moving parallel backward.

Section D

1–4: Move toward the right-hand side, watering the seeds with your hands in motion with the right hand over the left hand repeatedly for four counts. Move the legs in the same direction in a down/up motion.

5–8: Move toward the left-hand side, watering the seeds with your hands in motion with the right hand over the left repeatedly for four counts. Move legs in the same direction in a down/up motion.

Section E

Counterclockwise

1. Bend your body back as far as you can go and wiggle your entire body as you move for four counts counterclockwise.

Clockwise

2. Bend the body back as far as you can go and wiggle the entire body as you move for four counts clockwise.

FUBA

The rain dance called Fuba was introduced in Chapter 5.

Section A

Standing in place

Fuba begins with everyone clapping their hands in tune to the drums for 12 loud counts, starting from below with legs apart and clapping in between the legs, then up above the head.

Forward

1–8: Immediately after the claps, begin moving forward in a fast rhythmic drum movement, with hands rubbing against each other downward, then upward for eight counts forward.

Backward

9–16: Do the same movement backward, but rub your hands downward, then to the right and then again downward, then to the left for eight counts backward.

Section B

Forward

1–8: Run forward, again with legs right behind left, then left behind right in a fast motion, with arms opening outward toward the side of the body with palms open in eight counts.

Backward

9–16: Run backward with legs right behind left, then left behind right in a fast motion, with arms opening outward toward the side of the body with palms open in eight counts.

Section C

Counterclockwise

1. Moving counterclockwise, begin to take a very deep step outward; lift your arms up and outward as wide as possible for four counts.

Clockwise

2. Moving clockwise, begin to take a really deep step outward; lift your arms up and outward as wide as possible for four counts.

Repeat both movements for another four counts.

Section D

Forward

1–8: Run forward, lifting your feet high up behind your butt (boombsey); roll your arms right over the left while running forward for eight counts.

Backward

9–16: Twist your body backward and hop onto the heels, right and left in backward motion, with arms bent at the elbows and twisting the elbows for eight counts.

Section E

Forward

1–8: Move forward with pelvic pulses, right arm waving way out to the side and backward, then left arm waving way out to the side and backward, all for eight counts.

Backward

9–16: Move backward with butt (boombsey) pulses, with both arms bent beside your body in a fist, swaying the fist back and forth as the body moves and pulses backward, all for eight counts.

Section F

Counterclockwise

1. Begin to move counterclockwise around the room, stomping both feet into the ground in a fast "pita-pata" motion with both hands over your head, then down your shoulders, then down your entire body in a fast eight counts. After you touch right, open your palms wide face down beside your hips.

Clockwise

2. Begin to move clockwise around the room, stomping both feet into the ground in a fast "pita-pata" motion with both hands over your head, then down your shoulders, then down your entire body in a fast eight counts. After you touch right, open your palms wide face down beside your hips.

As you learn to navigate through these ten dances, you will realize they will become second nature to you. These ten dances presented in the Africa Dance I class at George Mason University will help you appreciate the rich history of the countries represented, as well as realize the importance of dance in African culture.

GLOSSARY

Cherie Nicaise	A beliefs and worship dance performed in reverence to both ancestors and other tribes for a pardon of something done wrong, or for a request of a favor needed
Dekonalan	A ceremonial dance performed during the time of seed sowing for the villages and townships in order for blessings to be received for their harvests
Djolo	A West African dance into manhood and womanhood
Freedom	A Zulu dance that signifies the bondage of the South Africans and their ensuing freedom
Fuba	Several tribal rain dances performed to their God so He may send down rain from above for their physical needs and everyday lives
Koumbe Oleli	A dance about warriors preparing for war that is performed by the West African people of Ghana, the Ashanti tribe
Ma Gaue	A West African births and ceremonies dance performed to their ancestors
M'buta Zao	A power and loyalty dance that originates from Cameroon and the Republic of the Congo.
Mystique	A central African dance about the mysteries of life
Somebody	A dance dating from the apartheid era, when the people of South Africa went through oppression and hard times

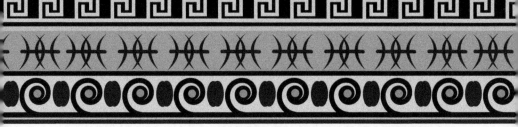

Chapter 7

HISTORY OF AFRICAN DANCE STYLES

HISTORICAL OVERVIEW OF AFRICAN DANCES

A historical overview of the dances in Africa are celebratory in nature. Africans brought their dances and music with them to America. Today, their influence and culture can still be seen in the performing arts of the Americans in dances such as step, tap, modern, interpretive, ballet, lyrical, break dancing, hip hop, jazz, and krumping.

The movements of the dances are sometimes natural imitations of animals, birds, reptiles, and wildlife. Daily work activities of the people that signify gracefulness, beauty, strength, bravery, and intelligence are also evident in certain dances. The rhythms of the drums are obtained from watching and studying the wonders of nature and the essence of life. The dances and the drumming are passed down from generation to generation to the children as early as the age of three when the child can comprehend.

Many of the African traditions, which were brought to America by way of the slaves—now even more so by voluntary visitors from Africa—are being kept alive through cultural dances and music taught to the American people by some of the natives of Africa.

Tribes play an integral part of the African people. Each region in a particular country is made up of several tribes. These tribes speak different languages or dialects, and each tribe practices different rituals and beliefs throughout the continent. This diversity accounts for the magnitude of the tribes and languages of the people of Africa.

In the continent of Africa, every country has a certain number of tribes, and each tribe performs its very own ceremonial dances; thus, each dance depicts the description of each race and tribe of that country. Dance is viewed as a way of life to the African people. Every occasion must be celebrated. Without second thought or planning, it becomes a party, regardless of the occasion. Everyone gets together, food is prepared, and music is played, and dancing begins. This can go on until daybreak. Unlike Western culture, there are usually no formal invitations to a party because everyone who is invited ends up bringing a couple of friends with them.

Ancestry

The historical overview of the dances shows they are to celebrate important events such as births and initiations, courtships and marriages, royalty and power, harvests and rituals, beliefs and worship, spirits and ancestors, and deaths and funerals.

Artists and choreographers take their work to heart back home, but because the artists are treated as part of the culture, the natives do not treat them as celebrities like the rest of the world does. It is taken for granted—and not rewarded—as it would be in the Western Hemisphere.

The dances are viewed as part of daily life. Africans will perform a dance for every occasion under the sun. Their culture is not complete without song and dance. That is the one thing no one can take away from Africans. One can see it during the time of the slave trade in America, as well as during apartheid in South Africa. The one thing that kept the Africans alive and sane was their music and dance, and that kept them together.

Ritual

Rituals are the traditional practices of the villages on the continent of Africa. Village life in Africa is totally different from city life, and every occasion is celebrated. From births and initiations, to courtships and marriages, to royalty and power, to harvests and rituals, to beliefs and worships, to spirits and ancestors, to deaths and burials, each calls for celebration. Although it may seem morbid to some cultures that funerals are celebrated, Africans believe in celebrating a life well lived. Births are as important as deaths to Africans. The importance of these dances and their cultural roots are what students of African dance will learn. African dance has retained its ritualistic character for centuries and was able to survive colonialism. Traditional dances among the tribes are mainly participatory in nature. The audience is always invited to join the performers, as they are all from the same community. Dance is used to interpret the meaning of certain rituals as well as ceremonies. Ritual dances symbolize the spirit of the individual in connection to the ancestors; therefore, it is a powerful format for keeping in touch with the spirit world. Since humans are viewed as spirits first before flesh, the ritual rite of passage is viewed as a journey of the spirit.

Ceremonial

Ceremonies are performed in the form of dance by males, females, and sometimes children, as an ancestral dance, event, or worship in reverence to both ancestors and other tribes. For instance, when a child is born in Africa, there has to be a naming ceremony, which takes place about two weeks after the child's birth; it is usually done very early in the morning before the sun rises. The ceremony is performed by an elder (in the true traditional sense) of the family, along with all the customary rights. This sort of ceremonial performance then turns into an all-day party as the invitees can drop by any time, regardless of the invited time, throughout the entire day. The food, music, and dance also continue and can be prolonged into the following day. There is a saying: "In Africa, any excuse for a party!" Ceremony is the form of celebrating the rite of passage from one stage of life to another. Ceremonial dances are usually joyous in nature and call for spectators to clap, ululate, stomp, and vocalize in response along with the dancers and drummers. In some parts of Africa, the dancers wear leg, wrist, and waist rattles to add to the enhancement of the music being performed.

Welsh wrote of ceremonial dances: "Marpu is a dance of the Gio people of Liberia and its function is to entertain chiefs and special guests during the dry season. Totogiri is a Yoruba dance from the village of Western-Pele in Owo district, Nigeria. The dance is performed at marriages and naming ceremonies. Bangumanga is a Ghanaian victory dance performed by the chief's children and wife for him at a ceremonial occasion."

Power and Loyalty

Men are the token heads of the families and possess the power to be in charge of the household for the caring and feeding of its members. This sort of power allows the women respect for their men. In return, the women play their roles in loyalty and obedience to their men. Compared to Western society, where either a man or woman can be the breadwinner of the family, the reverse is true in Africa. Most men are looked up to and expected to take care of the spouse and children, and the women are usually the homemakers. When it comes to dances of males and females, you can usually see the part that the males perform are very strong, masculine-type moves, different from the female dance parts that are more twisting and shaking in movement. Traditionally, African men are expected to dance, as well as learn to play the drums or other homemade instruments. Drummers are predominantly male in an African dance performance, but this does not mean that females cannot play the drums as well in all African cultures. In certain tribes, one can see the females joining the males in percussion.

Initiation

Initiation is the introduction of young lives into adult lives. It is a ritual that is performed for the young ones to teach them the correct cultural ways of life, which will benefit them in their lives. Initiation is a time for learning responsibilities and skills that will enable the youth to contribute to their communities. In each and every country, initiation represents a cultural passageway one must take in order to get the respect they deserve. In Ghana, one of the well-known initiations in the Ashanti region is called Bragoro, where females are initiated into womanhood before they get married. In the Akan culture, women are known to represent the beauty, purity, and dignity of the society and are guarded against corruption by going through this journey. When the girls are of age, under the supervision of an elderly woman in the community, they are taken to a designated place set aside for their training and the ushering of them into becoming reputable women.

Every young girl who comes of age is supposed to remain a virgin until the rites are performed. Girls who go contrary to this norm are not allowed to go through this journey, and according to the laws of the village, they can be banished from the village or become outcasts. At the end of this initiation journey, the girls are paraded through the village performing initiation dances to the young men as possible suitors, signifying the completion of the initiation. This ritual is not only for the purposes just stated, but also traditionally for training the youth to be active in their societies.

Harvesting

Planting- and harvesting-type dances are performed in respect to ancestors whom they believe have a much better connection to Mother Earth. Celebrations are a part of the livelihood of the people of Africa. As mentioned before in the earlier chapters, there are two seasons in sub-Saharan Africa, which are the wet and dry seasons. The seriousness of the dry season, which lasts anywhere from four to six months, can cause much harm to the crops, which then cannot produce any harvest for that season. This becomes a great problem for the farmers to have a successful harvest. The tribes have particular dances for such occasions that they perform to their ancestors, whom they believe can intercede on their behalf to ask their God for rain and for a good harvest.

The Past Interwoven into Dance

Dance is a form of art, as well as a way of life for the people of Africa. Dances were created from everyday activities such as religion, history, politics, sociology, culture, and more. Dances in precolonial and colonial times of the African people have been ritually connected; thus, certain ceremonies have had to be performed in connection with the dances. The dances we have in Africa go way back to our ancestors, who passed them down to us today. The influence of African dances today is strongly evident among the Africans in the Diaspora. Looking back at the clapping, shouting, yelling, and ecstatic body movements of the dancing in Africa, one can see the equivalent of this in the charismatic churches of today. From worship to celebrations to performances, African dance in the past is depicted in certain genres of dance today.

The Present Interwoven into Dance

Dances today continue to reflect cultural heritage: Hip hop, modern jazz, break dancing, popping, tap, krumping, reggae, soul, stepping, salsa, merengue, rock, creative, jazz, and contemporary. Take the meaning of contemporary dance, for instance, according to Felix Begho: "It may be taken to mean an approach to dance limited only by the movement capability and sensitivity of the performer, and the imagination, courage, and craft of the choreographer." Just as in African dance, it's all about feeling the beats of the drums, the music, and the rhythms and letting it all resonate into your body to allow you to dance from within.

Aesthetics of the Dance Form or Styles

Unlike Western dance forms, African dance forms and styles are unrefined and reflect a much more natural movement to the body. To begin with, dancing barefoot gives the dancer the rawness of dance style. Robert Farris Thompson states that, "Presentation is important in any style of dance. It holds an especially high importance in West African Dance styles. African dance is visually stimulating and capable of arousing emotional responses as well as visual ones. Aesthetic is a mode of intellectual energy when standards are applied to actual cases." The dances are very repetitive and viewed as part of daily life. The aesthetic form of African dance is its appearance and its content. As stated by Thompson, "moral perfection in the African aesthetic as articulated is the cornerstone to understanding the African aesthetics. Culture has a lot to do with African dance, as it is described as spiritual and holistic due to the fact that all aspects of life are integrated into the dance choreography. Life connects mind, body, spirit, and soul as such is the connection in African dance."

Common Movements within African Dances

In African dance, there are certain common movements that involve total isolation of the body. African dance requires about four to five components of the body to move at one time. The head almost always moves with the arms; the rib cage and shoulders move differently from the waist and the boombsey, the buttocks; and the legs are doing a totally different movement. Coordination plays a great role in African dance, but due to the breakdown of the dance movements, students can achieve these dances. The best way to learn the common movements of African dance is to first learn the leg steps, then add the arms, then the body, and lastly the head when you are comfortable enough to move it. The movements require flexibility, vibrancy, high intensity, speed, energy, and drive. The dance requires bare feet that signify the connection to Mother Earth. Attitude and personality are also considered a part of this genre of dance. The background stories exemplify the mood that the dancer should be in and the complexities of the dance.

Importance of the Head and Neck

Head movement is key to African dance. For starters, the head is the beginning of the body, and to be coined a dancer, one has to learn the head movements, along with the total body movements. Africans believe that dancing involves all parts of the body, from the head and neck all the way down to the feet. The dancer also uses her eyelids in dancing, particularly the Akan dance from Ghana, West Africa, called Adowa. In this dance, the dancer exercises the head and neck alone to the beat of the drums in between the dance performance and then introduces the body movements as well. In every African dance, the head and neck are a very important aspect. One can tell the difference with this dance, even by the head and neck, as most genres of dance in the West do not emphasize the head and neck the way African dance does. With some of the dance movements, one looks so awkward if and when they are not moving their head and neck. It completes the dance movement and makes it authentic. In some parts of the continent, other ethnic groups actually have a head dance that involves only the head being twirled around to the beat of the drums. It is amazing!

Boombsey Movement

The word "boombsey" is a Caribbean word that means buttocks. It is not an African word, but I use it because it's a nicer word to describe the rear end and it sounds funny to the students and puts a smile on their faces. The buttocks are another part of the body that is frequently used in African dance. It is predominantly used in West, central, South, and also North Africa. East Africans are known to use their shoulders more than the buttocks in most of their dances.

In West African dances, it is very rare not to see the buttocks—or boombsey—move. They move at a rapid and vigorous pace to the fast drum beats and shake and ripple at such an extreme speed that one would think the boombsey was going at a hundred miles per hour. This experienced way of moving one's boombsey is acquired at an early age in life. Both males and females are required to move their boombseys, and the intensity of it depends on the tribe and the particular dance.

A very vivid example is seen in the latest Broadway musical play *Fela!* which is about Fela Anikulapo Ransome-Kuti, a legendary African musician from Nigeria in the 1970s, whose real-life story portrays his Afrobeat music. This kind of music is mainly danced with the boombsey.

The history of African dance encompasses ritualistic movements that have stood the test of time through ancient, precolonial, and colonial times, as well as the present. African dances are interwoven with traditions and are present in every aspect of life. Whether it involves the harvest, ceremony, initiations, power and loyalty, or rituals, these dances complement the events in which they are presented. The history of these dances have been passed on through the ages and now influence some modern dances. As a student of African dance, you will experience the parallels of the past interwoven with the present.

GLOSSARY

Afrobeat	West African highlife music blended with American jazz, pop, and funk
Boombsey	Buttocks
Bragoro	An Akan initiation dance performed by young girls

Krumping   A form of street dance that is highly energetic and exaggerated

Popping   A form of street dance that involves the isolation of the entire body

Step   A dance that involves various dance steps coordinated with the hands.

Ululate   A form of noisemaking with the tongue and voice during dancing

REFERENCES

Thompson, R. F. (1974). African Art in Motion, UCLA Art Council (Berkeley and Los Angeles: University of California Press.

Welsh, K. (2004). *African dance*. Philadelphia: Chelsea House Publishers.

Welsh Asante, K. (Ed.) (with quote by Felix Begho) (1996). *African dance: an artistic historical and philosophical inquiry.* African World Press, Inc.

SUGGESTED READING LIST

African Dance and Cultural Perspectives. Hanna, J. L. (1965). African Dances as Education. *Impulse*, 48–52. Illustrated; includes bibliography.

African Dance Research: Past, Present and Future. (1980). *African Journal*, 11.1–2: 42–51.

Body Language: Dance Innovator Bill T. Jones Speaks His Mind–With His Body, That Is. (2000, December). *Dance Spirit*, p. 56.

Brunvald, J. (Ed.). (1996). *Breakdancing, American folklore: An encyclopedia*. New York: Garland, pp. 101–102.

Dance and Religion (overview). (2005). In Lindsay Jones, Ed., *The encyclopedia of religion* (2nd ed.). New York: Macmillan Co., pp. 2134–2143.

Dance, sex, and gender: Signs of identity, dominance, defiance, and desire. (1988). Chicago: University of Chicago Press.

Davis, C. (1998). *Dance Teacher Now*, 20(1): 50–51.

Eliade, M. (Ed.). Dance and Religion (Overview). (1987). In *The encyclopedia of religion* (Vol. 4). New York: Macmillan Co., pp. 203–212.

Eternal Enchantress: Debbie Allen Pushed the Envelope with Her Latest Dance Sensation. (2000). *Dance Spirit*, March, p. 94.

Field Research in Africa Dance: Opportunities and Utilities. (1968). *Ethnomusicology*, 12: 101–106. Synopsized as "Dance Field Research: Some Whys and African Wherefores." In Richard Bull, Ed.

Hanna, W. J. (1968). Heart Beat of Uganda. *African Arts*, 1(3): 42–45, 85.

Mazrui, A. (Ed.). (1977). African Dance and the Warrior Tradition. Journal of African and Asian Studies, 12: 1–2.

Research in dance: Problems and possibilities. (1968). New York: Committee on Research in Dance, pp. 82–84.

Rowe, P., & Stodelle, E. (Eds.). (1973). The Highlife: A West African Urban Dance. Dance Research Monograph. New York: Committee on Research in Dance, pp. 138–152.

Status of African Dance Studies. (1966). *Africa*, 36: 303–307.

West, G., & Blumberg, R. (Eds.). (1990). *Dance and women's protest in Nigeria and the United States, women and social protest.* New York: Oxford University Press, pp. 333–345.

Van Zile, J. (Ed.). (1975). *Dance in world cultures: Selected readings.* New York: MSS Information Corporation, pp. 164–177.

CREDITS

Figure 1.1: Source: http://commons.wikimedia.org/wiki/File:Map-Africa-Regions.svg. Copyright in the Public Domain.

Figure 3.1: Source: http://commons.wikimedia.org/wiki/File:Illu_vertebral_column.jpg. Copyright in the Public Domain.

Figure 3.2: Source: http://commons.wikimedia.org/wiki/File:BodyPlanes.jpg. Copyright in the Public Domain.

Figure 3.3: Source: http://commons.wikimedia.org/wiki/File:Illu_trunk_muscles.jpg. Copyright in the Public Domain.

Figure 3.4: Copyright © 2012 Depositphotos/AlienCat.

Figure 3.5: Copyright © 2013 Depositphotos/ingridat.

Figure 3.6: Copyright © 2014 Depositphotos/CLIPAREA.

Figure 3.7: Copyright © BodyHeal.com.au (CC BY-SA 4.0) at http://www.bodyheal.com.au/blog/iliotibial-band-syndrome-symptoms-causes-treatment.

Figure 3.8: Copyright © 2012 Depositphotos/galdzer.

Figure 3.9: Copyright © 2014 Depositphotos/anutuno.

Figure 3.10: Copyright © 2014 Depositphotos/anutuno.

Figure 3.11: Adapted from: Copyright © Harrygouvas (CC BY-SA 3.0) at http://commons.wikimedia.org/wiki/File:Shin_Splint_Syndrome.jpg

Figure 3.12: Copyright © 2011 Depositphotos/Krisdog.

Figure 3.13: Copyright © 2014 Depositphotos/anutuno.

Figure 3.14: Copyright © 2014 Depositphotos/CLIPAREA.

Figure 3.15: Copyright © 2013 Depositphotos/ingridat.

Figure 3.16: Copyright © 2011 Depositphotos/memitina.

Figure 4.1: Copyright © Wellcome Images (CC by 4.0) at http://commons.wikimedia.org/wiki/File:Zulu_witch_doctor_dancing,_South_Africa_Wellcome_M0002710.jpg.

Figure 4.4: Copyright © 2011 Depositphotos/mehmetcan.

Lightning Source UK Ltd.
Milton Keynes UK
UKHW022205220620
365402UK00008B/572